Contrac ......*...y*

*A Pocketbook for General Practitioners
and Practice Nurses*
Sixth edition

John Guillebaud
Emeritus Professor
Family Planning and
Reproductive Health,
University College London
UK

informa
healthcare

Sixth edition published in the United Kingdom in 2007 by Informa Healthcare, Telephone House, 69–77 Paul Street, London EC2A 4LQ. Informa Healthcare is a trading division of Informa UK Ltd. Registered Office: 37/41 Mortimer Street, London W1T 3JH. Registered in England and Wales number 1072954.

Tel: +44 (0)20 7017 5000
Fax: +44 (0)20 7017 6336
Website: www.informahealthcare.com

First published in the United Kingdom in 1992 as *Contraception: Hormonal and Barrier Methods* by Martin Dunitz, an imprint of the Taylor & Francis Group plc, 11 New Fetter Lane, London EC4P 4EE

This book represents the personal opinions of John Guillebaud, based wherever possible on published and sometimes unpublished evidence. When (as is not infrequent) no epidemiological or other direct evidence is available, clinical advice herein is always as practical and realistic as possible and based, pending more data, on the author's judgement of other sources. These may include the opinions of Expert Committees and any existing Guidelines. In some instances the advice appearing in this book may even so differ appreciably from the latter, for reasons usually given in the text and (since medical knowledge and practice are continually evolving) relates to the date of publication. Healthcare professionals must understand that they take ultimate responsibility for their patient and ensure that any clinical advice they use from this book is applicable to the specific circumstances that they encounter.

A CIP record for this book is available from the British Library.

ISBN 978 0 415 41743 3

Distributed in North and South America by
Taylor & Francis
6000 Broken Sound Parkway, NW, (Suite 300)
Boca Raton, FL 33487, USA

Within Continental USA
Tel: 1 (800) 272 7737; Fax: 1 (800) 374 3401
Outside Continental USA
Tel: (561) 994 0555; Fax: (561) 361 6018
Email: ordrs@crcpress.com

Distributed in the rest of the world by
Thomson Publishing Services
Cheriton House
North Way
Andover, Hampshire SP10 5BE, UK
Tel.: +44 (0)1264 332424
E-mail: tps.tandfsalesorder@thomson.com

Composition by Scribe Design Ltd, Ashford, Kent, UK
Printed and bound in India by Replika Press Pvt Ltd

Statement of competing interests
The author has received payments for research projects, lectures, *ad hoc* consultancy work and related expenses from the manufacturers of contraceptive products.

Contents

Preface   iv

Acknowledgements   iv

Introduction   1

Combined hormonal contraception   11

Progestogen-only pill   68

Injectables   80

Contraceptive implants   90

Intrauterine contraception   98

Postcoital contraception   124

Other reversible methods   134

Special considerations   144
   Exclusion of pregnancy   144
   Contraception for the older woman   146

Appendix   150
   Use of licensed products in an
     unlicensed way   150
   Believable websites in reproductive health   152
   Further reading   153
   Glossary   154

Index   157

Preface

'... how successful we have beome. We as a species together with our cows, pigs etc, we are about 97 per cent of the biomass of all veretebrate species, meaning only 3 per cent are wild species'.

Mathis Wackernagel, in The Ecological Footprint, 2005

We have not inherited the earth from our grandparents, we have borrowed it from our grandchildren.

Kashmiri proverb

Family planning could bring more benefits to more people at less cost than any other single technology now available to the human race.

James Grant, UNICEF, 1992

Climate change increases with growth in the numbers of climate changERS More Humanity with fewer Humans (through voluntary contraception)

Slogans of the Optimum Population Trust, 2006

Born and reared in Burundi and Rwanda, countries whose recurrent agonies are in significant measure related to excessive population growth, I maintain that:

Human **needs** along with those of all other species with which we share the Natural World will never be sustainably met on a finite planet without more concerned, non-coercive, action on human **numbers**.

No woman on earth who at time present wishes to exercise her human right to have control of her fertility should be denied the means to do so, by barriers produced by any agency – whether through her partner's refusal, her society's pro-natalism, misinformation (sometimes deliberate), or lack of available, affordable and accessible contraceptive supplies and services.

In their life-time, every new birth in the UK will, through the inevitable effluence of his or her affluence as a consumer, harm the environment – by climate change and in numerous other ways – as much as 30, or on some criteria 200, births in Burundi or Bangladesh will ever do. We all have a part to play in ensuring that our grandchildren receive back their 'loan' in a halfway decent and long-term sustainable state (see www.ecotimecapsule.com). As a small but relevant contribution to that endeavour, I welcome this opportunity to bring a new edition of this pocketbook on contraception to general practioners and nurses in Primary Care.

I write, moreover, as one who is proud to have worked in general practice, as a locum in places as diverse as Barnsley, Cambridge, Luton and South London, and hence able to appreciate some of the satisfactions and the constraints of that role.

John Guillebaud. May 2007

Acknowledgements
I wish to thank numerous friends and colleagues in the UK and abroad working in relevant specialist and general practice – too many to mention all by name. Toni Belfield, Head of Information at the UK FPA, Dr Anne MacGregor, MPC's Medical Adviser, and Alison Campbell, Ian Mellor and Robert Peden of the Informa Healthcare Imprint who have guided this work now through five editions, do however deserve special mention. I acknowledge much help recently from Susan Brechin and staff of the Clinical Effectiveness Unit of the Faculty of Family Planning and Reproductive Health Care (FFPRHC) and, over many years, from senior medical and nursing staff at the Margaret Pyke Centre (MPC) and Oxford Family Planning Clinics; and I am also grateful to some of our clients for the insights they have given me.

John Guillebaud is Emeritus Professor of Family Planning and Reproductive Health at University College London, Honorary Consultant in Reproductive Health for the Oxford Community Primary Care Trust, and Surgeon and Research Director at the Elliot-Smith Vasectomy Clinic, Churchill Hospital, Oxford.

Until 2002, he was also Medical Director of the Margaret Pyke Centre in London, and continues as a Trustee of the Margaret Pyke Memorial Trust.

Introduction

General practitioners (GPs) and practice nurses are often best placed to offer good contraceptive advice because they already know the patient's health and family circumstances. Some practices are excellent; others provide little beyond oral contraception and devote insufficient time and skill to counselling. The 2002 Sexual Health Strategy established that primary care should always supply at least Level 1 basic contraceptive services, and should consider also supplying services at Level 2. These include all the long-acting reversible contraceptive methods (LARCs). The National Institute for Health and Clinical Excellence (NICE) Clinical Guideline No. 30 (www.nice.org.uk, 2005) drew attention to the many contraceptive (and sometimes non-contraceptive) advantages of these, comprising injectables, implants, the latest copper-banded intrauterine devices (IUDs) and the levonorgestrel intrauterine system (LNG IUS). If not supplied on site, practices should have straightforward referral arrangements in place for the LARCs, and also when appropriate for Level 3 services such as male and female sterilization, and legal abortion.

Iatrogenic ('doctor-caused') pregnancies are a reality. They result from avoidable errors or omissions on the part of service providers: especially, the omission of sufficient *time* for the consultation. Women choosing their first-ever 'medical' contraceptive need more time than the usual 10 minutes available in most surgeries. Indeed, the *National Service Standards Framework* recommends 'At least 20 minutes should be allocated to a practitioner or clinical team (e.g. nurse and doctor) for ... a new consultation' (UK National Service Standard, 2005 www.ffprhc.org.uk/admin/uploads/ServiceStandards forWorkloadFINAL.pdf): 20 minutes is very daunting yet not actually unreasonable, when one considers the ground to be covered say for a first-time pill-user (see p. 55). An arrangement that works well in some practices is to offer routinely a second 10–15 minute consultation within the same week, at the end of a surgery or with the practice nurse.

Much of this work can – indeed should – be delegated to a practice nurse fully trained in family planning, usually with a gain rather than a loss in standards. Practice is changing fast, with more use of patient group directions and more trained nurses who are prescribers and practitioners, some of whom insert intrauterine and subdermal contraceptives. Aside from those, a good mainstream practice nurse may appropriately perform the following delegated functions:

- Taking sexual and medical history, discussion of choices (using UK Family Planning Association (FPA) leaflets)
- Cap fitting, checking, teaching
- Pill teaching
- Pill issuing/reissuing and emergency pill issuing – given fully agreed and audited patient group directions
- Pill monitoring, including migraine assessment and blood pressure (BP)
- Contraceptive injections: depot medroxyprogesterone acetate (DMPA; Depo-Provera, Pharmacia & Upjohn)
- IUD and IUS checks, including eliciting cervical excitation tenderness
- Cervical smear taking

Formal training is also desirable for doctors,* and should include both theoretical and 'apprenticeship' training, as well as discussion of the often complex psychosexual and emotional factors involved in the use of contraception. All clinicians should be sensitive to hidden signals in this area.

* In the UK, the Faculty of Family Planning and Reproductive Health Care (FFPRHC – in this book termed 'the Faculty of FP') offers, through agencies such as the Margaret Pyke Centre (MPC), educational courses for doctors leading to their Diploma (DFFP) and Membership (MFFP), as well as Letters of Competence in Intrauterine Techniques, Subdermal Implants and Instructing. In 2002, nurses and associate practitioners working in reproductive health became eligible to become Associates of the Faculty. The Institute of Psychosexual Medicine and the British Association for Sexual and Relationship Therapy also offer relevant training courses and seminars (websites on p. 152).

Doctors or nurses should back their counselling with good literature. Although some manufacturers have improved their package labelling, the latest FPA leaflets are better – user-friendly, yet accurate and comprehensive. The one called *Your Guide to Contraception* tabulates all the important methods, both reversible and permanent, and is ideal for reading in the waiting room before counselling. The leaflets on individual methods should be given with advice to 'read, and keep long term for further reference'. The month and date of publication should be recorded in the patient's notes. Follow-up patients may need a replacement. Together with accurate contemporary records, these leaflets provide strong medicolegal back-up for practitioners who may be asked to justify their actions in the event of litigation. They are an essential supplement to – but by no means a replacement for – time spent with the health care practitioner.

Choice of method

Most women who seek contraception are healthy and young, and present fewer problems than the over-35s, teenagers and those with intercurrent disease. There is a tendency for sterilization procedures to be demanded at too early an age. This is partly because the Pill is too often seen as synonymous with contraception, and we as providers have not been informing women about the many new or improved reversible alternatives, about which there is still much mythology and ignorance. See Figure 1: the methods at bottom left are known collectively as the LARCs – the levonorgestrel IUS (LNG-IUS), the banded copper IUDs, injectables and the latest implants. All of these, while being reversible, have efficacy of the very same order as female sterilization.

The young

I am opposed to 'sex education'! What we should all favour, and promote, is sex *and relationships* education (SRE). When seeking advice on sex, relationships, contraception, pregnancy and parenthood, young people are entitled to accessible, confidential, non-judgemental and unbiased support and guidance – recognizing the diversity of their cultural and faith traditions. We

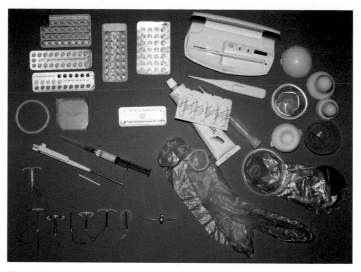

Figure 1
The choice of methods in the UK. (Reproduced with kind permission of Dr Anne MacGregor.)

should listen to their views and respect their opinions and choices. Valid choices include waiting (not yet having) as well as having (safer and contracepted) sex.

However, as they may often 'get away with it' in one or more cycles, all too often the young do not seek advice until they have already conceived. Easier access to emergency contraception is an obvious priority. But education must promote (as in the Netherlands) the societal norm that sex may be a feature of a good relationship only when and if adequate contraception exists. In this age group, we still await as first-line more 'forget-table' methods in which (in contrast to the Pill) non-pregnancy is the default state. Injectables and implants are usually prefer-able to copper IUDs although these are only relatively contraindicated (WHO 3 or even WHO 2 in true mutual monogamy). The LNG-IUS may also be appropriate.

With young people under 16 years of age, it remains logical – so long as it is done opportunely, non-judgementally and never in a patronizing way – to present the emotional, physical and legal advantages of delaying coitarche and then of mutually faithful relationships. But even if that is medically the 'best', when rejected it must not become the enemy of the 'good', a category that surely includes contraception combined with age-appropriate SRE – which ideally should be started at home by the parent(s) and not just left to schools. Legally, following the Guidance below, in the decision to prescribe a medical method of contraception an attempt should first be made to involve a parent. Yet it can be good practice to initiate the Pill, say, or an injectable in the absence of such parental support.

- *At all times, the young woman must be assured of confidentiality* (this should be cast-iron – and feel so to her).
- Be alert for the possibility of sexual abuse – and if it ever becomes necessary for others to become involved (e.g. because abuse is indeed suspected), always inform the young person.
- Remember always the conclusion of a focus group of sexually active teens, in which they were asked 'Who would you like to help you with contraception?'... their response was 'Someone with a smile would be your best bet'. This speaks volumes about their past experience.

There is a useful mnemonic for the 'Fraser guidelines' regarding under-16s (UK Memorandum of Guidance: DHSS HC(FP)86) that still applies, though issued shortly after the Gillick case in 1985.

Mnemonic: UnProtected SSexual interCourse. The health care practitioner:

U Must ensure the young person **UNDERSTANDS** the potential risks and benefits of the treatment/advice given

P Is legally obliged to discuss the value of **PARENTAL** support, yet the client must know that confidentiality is respected whether or not this is given

S Should assess whether the client is likely to have **SEXUAL** intercourse without contraception

S Should assess whether the young person's physical/mental health may **SUFFER** if not given contraceptive advice or supplies

I Must consider if it is in the client's best **INTERESTS** to give contraception without parental consent

C Must respect the duty of **CONFIDENTIALITY** that should be given to a person under 16, and which is as great as that owed to any other person

If the above Guidance is followed in utmost good faith, the prescription of a medical method of contraception will never be seen in Law as aiding or abetting the commission of any crime.

Sexually transmitted infections

Taking a quick but matter-of-fact sexual history need not be stressful. It should be seen as part of the consultation for *all* contraceptives, not just the intrauterine ones. Ask:

- 'When did you last have sex?' and then immediately
- 'When did you last have sex with anybody different?'

Much can be learnt from the second of this pair of open questions, whether the response is 'about 21 years ago'... or '3 months ago'. If the latter, it is now unthreatening to go on and clarify whether this was a change of partner or 'a one night stand' – and whether there have been others in the past year. Getting a handle on whether the woman's partner himself is monogamous or otherwise can be much more difficult (p. 109).

In the UK, *'higher risk' of infection* particularly with *Chlamydia trachomatis*, applies to women with:

- Age under 25, but a good history taken as above offers more discrimination, namely
- A partner change in the previous 12 weeks
- More than one partner in the past 12 months

Advise all about minimizing their risk of sexually transmitted infections (STIs), including HIV. If when counselling an individual the 'selling' of monogamy fails, *it is essential to promote the condom as an addition to their selected contraceptive, whenever (now or later) there may be an infection risk – the so-called 'Double-Dutch' approach.*

Features of the ideal contraceptive

- 100% effective (with the default state as contraception)
- 100% convenient (forgettable, non-coitally related)
- 100% safe, free of adverse side effects (neither risk nor nuisance)
- 100% reversible, ideally by self
- 100% maintenance-free, meaning it needs absolutely no

No available method meets all the criteria in the above box, though the LNG-IUS gets closest.

Relative effectiveness of the available methods

Failure rates of methods are usually expressed as per 100 woman-years. A figure of 10 per 100 woman-years for a 'perfect user' (see below) means that in a population of 100 users 10 women might be expected to conceive in the first year of use of the method; or, notionally, one woman would have an 'evens' chance of having an unplanned pregnancy after 10 years of its use. In Table 1, 'Perfect use' means the method is used both consistently and correctly, whereas 'Typical' use means what it says and is obviously hugely dependent on characteristics (e.g. age, social class, acceptability of conception, etc.) of the population studied. Note the huge difference in percentage conceiving after 1 year between the two types of use for the combined pill (0.3 versus 8). The data in this table come from the USA, but the 'Perfect use' data are usable for comparing methods in any setting.

Continuation rates also vary even among 'perfect' users and in general are much higher for the long-acting reversible methods.

Eligibility criteria for contraceptives

The World Health Organization system for classifying contraindications

This excellent scheme (first devised in a small WHO Workshop that I attended in 1994, in Atlanta) is more fully described in the

Table 1

Percentage of women experiencing an unintended pregnancy during the first year of use (data from USA)[a]

Contraceptive method	Percentage of women experiencing an unintended pregnancy within 1st year of use	
	Typical use	Perfect use
No method	85	85
Spermicides	29	18
Withdrawal	27	4
Periodic abstinence	25	
Calendar		9
Ovulation method		3
Sympto-thermal[b]		2
Post-ovulation		1
Cap plus spermicide		
Parous women	32	26
Nulliparous women	16	9
Sponge		
Parous women	32	20
Nulliparous women	16	9
Diaphragm	16	6
Condom		
Female	21	5
Male	15	2
Combined pill and minipill	8	0.3
Combined hormonal patch (Evra)	8	0.3
Combined hormonal ring (NuvaRing)	8	0.3
DMPA (Depo-Provera)	3	0.3
Combined injectable (Lunelle)	3	0.05
IUD		
ParaGard (banded copper T)[c]	0.8	0.6
Mirena (LNG-IUS)	0.1	0.1
LNG implants[d] (Norplant and Norplant-2)	0.05	0.05
Female sterilization	0.5	0.5
Male sterilization	0.15	0.10

Emergency contraceptive pills: Treatment initiated within 72 hours after unprotected intercourse reduces the risk of pregnancy by at least 75%.
Lactational amenorrhoea method: LAM is a highly effective, *temporary* method of contraception.

[a]Adapted from: *Medical Eligibility Criteria for Contraceptive Use* (WHOMEC), 3rd edn. Geneva: WHO, 2004. Data from: Trussell J. Contraceptive efficacy. In: Hutcher RA, Trussell J, Stewart F et al, eds. *Contraceptive Technology*, 18th rev edn. New York: Ardent Media, 2004.
[b]I.e. the cervical mucus method supplemented by calendar calculation in the pre-ovulatory phase and basal body temperature charting in the post-ovulatory phase. See p. 141.
[c]Equivalent to the T-Safe Cn380A (and its clones).
[d]Implanon has similar efficacy.

document issued by WHO, *Medical Eligibility Criteria for Contraceptive Use*, 3rd edn (Geneva: WHO, 2004), which will be referred to from now on as WHOMEC. This is dark blue in colour and its companion volume (green) is *Selected Practice Recommendations for Contraceptive Use* (Geneva: WHO, 2005), generally referred to as WHOSPR. Readily downloadable from www.who.int/reproductive-health (click 'family planning' and go to either medical eligibility criteria or selected practice recommendations), both of the documents are fully evidence-based, where evidence exists.

The FFPRHC's Clinical Effectiveness Unit has since developed a UK version (UKMEC) of WHOMEC, which adjusts for UK practice and so differs slightly – therefore in most (but not quite all) cases being more closely congruent with this book. UKMEC is available on the FFPRHC website: www.ffprhc.org.uk.

Both WHOMEC AND UKMEC classify eligibility for contraceptive methods into four categories, as in the following box:

WHO Classification of contraindications
(A–D is the author's parallel aide-memoire for the significance of each caegory)
1. A condition for which there is no restriction for the use of the contraceptive method
   'A' is for **Always Usable**
2. A condition where the advantages of the method generally outweigh the theoretical or proven risks
   'B' is for **Broadly Usable, Be alert** (for any future added risk)

* * * * *

3. A condition where the theoretical or proven risks usually outweigh the advantages, so an alternative method is usually preferred. Yet, respecting the patient/client's autonomy, if she accepts the risks and rejects or should not use relevant alternatives, given the risks of pregnancy the method can be used with caution/sometimes with additional monitoring
   'C' is for **'Caution/Counselling'**, if used at all
4. A condition that represents an unacceptable health risk
   'D' is for **'DO NOT USE'**, at all

The most useful new feature of the classification is the separation into two categories of 'Relative' contraindication (WHO 2 and 3), with the 'strong relative' ones (WHO 3) *below the line*: implying that they *normally indicate non-use* of the method.

Clinical judgement is required, always in consultation with the contraceptive user, especially (1) in all WHO 3 conditions or (2) if more than one condition applies. As a working rule, two WHO 2 conditions move the situation to WHO 3; and if any WHO 3 condition applies, the addition of either a 2 or a 3 condition normally means WHO 4, i.e. 'Do not use'.

For all the medical methods described in the rest of this book, the listed absolute or relative contraindications are based on the WHOMEC scheme. Given that prescribers often have to make a decision (in consultation with the woman/couple) despite a frustrating absence of good evidence, pending more data, what follows is the best interim guidance, according to this author's judgement of the evidence. This is often because the WHO has not as yet given its verdict on many issues – although where it has, the category here is generally the same as in WHOMEC and UKMEC: if not, attention is drawn to the difference.

Combined hormonal contraception

COMBINED ORAL CONTRACEPTIVES

Mechanism of action

The combined oral contraceptive (COC) pills currently available in the UK are shown in Table 2. They combine an estrogen (ethinylestradiol (EE) in all cases but one) with one of seven progestogens.

Aside from secondary contraceptive effects on the cervical mucus and to impede implantation, COCs primarily prevent ovulation. This makes the method highly effective in 'perfect' use (Table 1), but it removes the normal menstrual cyle and replaces it with a cycle that is user-produced and based only on the end-organ, i.e. the endometrium. So the withdrawal bleeding has minimal medical significance, can be deliberately postponed or made infrequent (e.g. tricycling, discussed below), and if it fails to occur, once pregnancy is excluded, poses no problem. The pill-free time is the contraception-deficient time, which has great relevance to advice for the maintenance of COC efficacy (see below).

Benefits versus risks

Capable of providing virtually 100% protection from unwanted pregnancy and taken at a time unconnected with sexual activity, the COC provides enormous reassurance by the associated regular, short, light and usually painless withdrawal bleeding at the end of the 21-day pack. Inevitably, most of this section will

Table 2 Formulations of currently marketed combined oral contraceptives (COCs)[a]

Pill type	Preparation	Estrogen (µg)	Progestogen (µg)
Monophasic			
Ethinylestradiol/ norethisterone type	Loestrin 20	20	1000 Norethisterone acetate[b]
	Loestrin 30	30	1500 Norethisterone acetate[b]
	Brevinor	35	500 Norethisterone
	Ovysmen	35	500 Norethisterone
	Norimin	35	1000 Norethisterone
Ethinylestradiol/ levonorgestrel	Microgynon 30 (also ED)	30	150
	Ovranette	30	150
Ethinylestradiol/ desogestrel	Mercilon	20	150
	Marvelon	30	150
Ethinylestradiol/ gestodene	Femodette	20	75
Ethinylestradiol/ gestodene	Femodene (also ED)	30	75
	Minulet	30	75
Ethinylestradiol/ norgestimate	Cilest	35	250
Ethinylestradiol drospirenone	Yasmin	30	3000
Mestranol/ norethisterone	Norinyl-1	50	1000
Bi/triphasic			
Ethinylestradiol/ norethisterone	BiNovum	35 / 35	500 } 833[c] (7 tabs) / 1000 (14 tabs)
	Synphase	35 / 35 / 35	500 (7 tabs) / 1000 } 714 (9 tabs) / 500 (5 tabs)
	TriNovum	35 / 35 / 35	500 (7 tabs) / 750 } 750 (7 tabs) / 1000 (7 tabs)
Ethinylestradiol/ levonorgestrel	Logynon (also ED)	30 / 40 } 32[c] / 30	50 (6 tabs) / 75 } 92 (5 tabs) / 125 (10 tabs)
	Trinordiol	30 / 40 } 32 / 30	50 (6 tabs) / 75 } 92 (5 tabs) / 125 (10 tabs)
Ethinylestradiol/ gestodene	Tri-Minulet	30 / 40 } 32 / 30	50 (6 tabs) / 70 } 79 (5 tabs) / 100 (10 tabs)
	Triadene	30 / 40 } 32 / 30	50 (6 tabs) / 70 } 79 (5 tabs) / 100 (10 tabs)
Ethinylestradiol/ cyproterone acetate	Dianette[d]	35	2000

[a]Other names in use worldwide are on the website www.ippf.org.uk.
[b]Converted to norethisterone as the active metabolite.
[c]Equivalent daily doses for comparison with monophasic brands.
[d]Marketed primarily as acne therapy (see text), and not intended to be used as a routine pill.

be on possible risks and hazards associated with taking the Pill, but the positive aspects should not be forgotten; they are listed in the second box below. Although some of these findings await full confirmation, the good news is rarely mentioned while the suspected risks are widely publicized and often over-dramatized.

Space does not allow full discussion of all the work that has been published in the 45 years during which the Pill has been available in this country. Practitioners should form their own opinion of the risks and benefits by their own reading, but the following may help to summarize present medical opinion upon which contemporary prescription of the Pill is based.

The data presented here have been derived mainly from the prospective Royal College of General Practitioners (RCGP), Oxford/FPA and US Nurses Studies, supplemented by numerous case–control studies and a few randomised controlled trials conducted by the WHO and other bodies.

Contraceptive benefits of COCs
- Effectiveness
- Convenience, not intercourse related
- Reversibility

Non-contraceptive benefits of COCs
These at times may provide the principal indication for use of the method (e.g. in the treatment of dysmenorrhoea in a not-yet sexually active teenager)
- Reduction of most menstrual cycle disorders: less heavy bleeding, therefore less anaemia, and less dysmenorrhoea; regular bleeding, the timing of which can be controlled (no Pill taker need have 'periods' at weekends; upon request, she may tricycle and so bleed only a few times a year); fewer symptoms of premenstrual tension overall; no ovulation pain
- Reduced risk of cancers of ovary and endometrium (see text), and very possibly also colorectal cancer
- Fewer functional ovarian cysts, because abnormal ovulation is prevented
- Fewer extrauterine pregnancies, because normal ovulation is inhibited
- Reduction in pelvic inflammatory disease (PID)
- Reduction in benign breast disease
- Fewer symptomatic fibroids

- Probable reduction in thyroid disease, whether over- or under-active
- Probable reduction in risk of rheumatoid arthritis
- Fewer sebaceous disorders, especially acne (with estrogen-dominant COCs such as Marvelon™ and Yasmin™)
- Possible reduced risk of endometriosis (a potential benefit probably not as well realised as it would be if the Pill were taken in a bleed-free regimen)
- Continuous use beneficial in long-term suppression of endometriosis
- Possibly fewer duodenal ulcers (not well established)
- Reduction in *Trichomonas vaginalis* infections
- Possible lower incidence of toxic shock syndrome
- No toxicity in overdose
- Some obvious beneficial social effects, to balance suggested negatives

Even as we turn to unwanted effects, it is reassuring that, according to the RCGP report in 1999, COCs have their main (small) effect on every known associated cause of mortality during current use and for some (variable) time thereafter. The excess thrombotic risk has probably vanished by 4 weeks, and by 10 years after use ceases, mortality in past-users is indistinguishable from that in never-users.

Tumour risk and COCs

No medication continues to receive so much scrutiny and investigation as the Pill. For some time, fears have been expressed about its possible connection with breast, cervical and liver cancers.

Breast cancer

The incidence of this disease is high, and therefore it must inevitably be expected to develop in women whether they take COCs or not. Since the recognized risk factors include early menarche and late age of first birth, use by young women was rightly bound to receive scientific scrutiny. The literature to date is copious, complex, confusing and contradictory!

The 1996 publication by the Collaborative Group on Hormonal Factors in Breast Cancer reanalysed original data relating to over 53 000 women with breast cancer and over 100 000 controls from 54 studies in 25 countries. This is 90% of the world epidemiological data. The reanalysis showed disappearance of the risk in ex-users, but recency of use of the COC was shown to be the most important factor: with the odds ratio unaffected by age of initiation or discontinuation, use before or after first full-term pregnancy, or duration of use. The main findings are summarized in Table 3 and below. A 2002 study of 4575 breast cancer patients and matched cancer-free controls in the USA was congruent with this and particularly reassuring in that there was nothing to suggest the so-called 'time-bomb': despite 75% exposure to the COC in the population, there was *no persistence of risk in long-time ex-users* when they reached ages with much higher incidence of this cancer, as shown in Figure 2.

Table 3
The increased risk of developing breast cancer while taking the pill and in the 10 years after stopping[a]

User status	Increased risk
Current user	24%
1–4 years after stopping	16%
5–9 years after stopping	7%
10 plus years an ex-user	No significant excess

[a]Collaborative Group on Hormonal Factors in Breast Cancer. *Lancet* 1996; **347**: 1713–27.

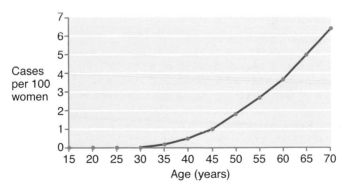

Figure 2
Background risk: cumulative number of breast cancers per 100 women, by age. (Reproduced from statement by Faculty of Family Planning, June 1996.)

COC-users can be reassured that:

- While the small increase in breast cancer risk for women on the Pill noted in previous studies is confirmed, the odds ratio of 1.24 signifies an increase of 24% only while women are taking the COC, diminishing to zero after discontinuation, over the next few years.
- Beyond 10 years after stopping, there is no detectable increase in breast cancer risk for former Pill-users.
- The cancers diagnosed in women who use or have ever used COCs are clinically less advanced than those who have never used the Pill, and are less likely to have spread beyond the breast.
- These risks are not associated with duration of use, or the dose or type of hormone in the COC, and there is no synergism with other risk factors for breast cancer (e.g. family history).
- If 1000 women use the pill till age 35, by age 45 this model shows there will be, in all, 11 cases of breast cancer. Importantly, however, as portrayed in Figure 3, only one of these cases is extra (i.e. pill-related), the others would have arisen anyway, in a control group of 1000 never-users.

Clinical implications

The breast cancer issue should now normally be addressed, in a sensitive way, as part of routine Pill counselling for all women. This discussion should be initiated opportunely – not necessarily at the first visit if not raised by the woman – along with encouragement to report promptly any unusual changes in their breasts at any time in the future ('breast awareness'). The balancing protective effects against at least two malignancies (ovary and endometrium: see below) should also be mentioned. The known contraceptive and non-contraceptive benefits of COCs may seem so great to many (but not to all) as to compensate for almost any likely lifetime excess risk of breast cancer.

- *What about Pill use by the older women?* There is no change in relative risk, but an increased attributable risk (3 extra cases per 1000 for 10th year ex-users now aged 55, instead of the above 1 extra case per 1000 for 10th year ex-users now 45). This must be explained and may be acceptable to many, given the balancing (see below) from the established protection against cancer of the ovary and endometrium – whose risks also increase with age. But these data about the COC combined with new choices now available should lead to more older women choosing other contraceptive options (such as the IUD or IUS; see below).

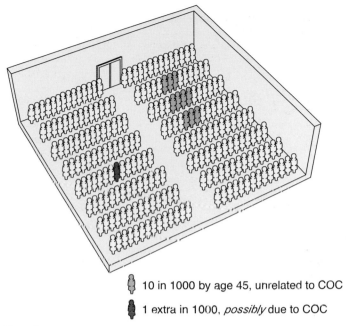

🧍 10 in 1000 by age 45, unrelated to COC

🧍 1 extra in 1000, *possibly* due to COC

Figure 3
Cumulative incidence of breast cancer during and after use of COC until age 35.

- Women with benign breast disease (BBD) or with a *family history of a young first-degree relative with breast cancer under age 40* have a larger background risk than the generality of women – but only the same as women slightly older than their current age who are free of the risk factor. UKMEC classifies both of these conditions as WHO 1 for the COC (no restriction on use).
- *If the woman with BBD had a breast biopsy*, the histology should be obtained: if epithelial atypia (pre-malignant) was found, the situation for the COC changes to WHO 4.
- *Carriers of known gene mutations* (e.g. *BRCA1*) associated with this cancer should normally avoid the COC (WHO 3).
- *If a woman develops carcinoma of the breast*, COCs should be discontinued, and women with a personal history of this cancer should avoid COCs (WHO 4). UKMEC, like WHOMEC, allows COC use after 5 years of remission.

We can be sure that the last word has not yet been spoken on this issue of breast cancer and the Pill.

Cervical cancer

Studies of cervical cancer are complicated by lack of accurate information on sexual activity of women and especially their partners. Human papillomavirus (HPV) types 16 and 18 are important candidates as the principal carcinogen, which is clearly transmitted sexually. Review of the studies – including those that identified and controlled for the presence of HPV – leads to the conclusion that the COC acts as a cofactor, speeding transition through the stages of cervical intraepithelial neoplasia (CIN). The raised odds ratio is clearly increased with increasing durations of use, and may persist in ex-users. In this respect, it is similar to, but certainly weaker than, cigarette smoking.

Clinical implications
- Prescribers must ensure that COC-users and ex-users are adequately screened following agreed guidelines. Even if they also smoke, a 3-yearly smear frequency starting from age 25, as in national guidelines, is still believed to suffice to identify – and then treat appropriately – the vast majority – though not all – in pre-invasive stages, before actual cancer develops.
- It is acceptable practice (WHO 2) to continue COC use during the careful monitoring of any abnormality, or after definitive treatment of CIN.

Liver tumours

COC use increases the relative risk of *benign adenoma* or *hamartoma*, either of which can cause pain or rarely a haemoperitoneum. However, the background incidence is so small (1–3 per 1 million women per year) that the COC-attributable risk is minimal. Most reported cases have been in long-term users of relatively high-dose pills. Three case–control studies also support the view that the rare *primary hepatocellular carcinoma* is minimally less rare in COC users than it is in controls. Yet there is reassuring contrary evidence that, although this cancer is usually rapidly fatal, the attributable death rate has not changed detectably in the USA or Sweden, where the COC has been widely used since the 1960s. Moreover there is no evidence of synergism with either cirrhosis or hepatitis B liver infection.

Clinical implications
A past history of tumour (benign or malignant) is WHO 4 for the COC but WHO 3 for other forms of hormonal contraception (WHOMEC).

Choriocarcinoma or, more generally, all gestational trophoblastic disease

In the presence of active trophoblastic disease, early studies from the UK showed that chemotherapy for choriocarcinoma was more often required among women given COCs. This has not been shown in studies from the USA – probably because chemotherapy there is given to almost all cases of trophoblastic disease, thereby obliterating any hormonal effect. There remains a theoretical risk that the COC may promote metastatic disease or drug-resistant disease.

Despite WHOMEC classifying any form of trophoblastic disease as WHO 1, it is still recommended by UKMEC and the UK regional centres monitoring all UK cases that, so long as human chorionic gonadotrophin (hCG) levels are raised, COC should be avoided (WHO 4). *But thereafter, the COC is WHO 1, with no restriction on use.*

Clinical implications

- Women are advised not to conceive
  - for 6 months after hCG levels are normal, and
  - for at least 12 months from conclusion of any chemotherapy (because of a risk of recurrent disease and teratogenic effects of the chemotherapy).
- So what contraception should be used?
  - Fortunately, while hCG levels are above 5000 IU/l, ovulation is very improbable, so barrier methods should be effective and these are first choice for what is usually a short time.
  - The progestogen-only methods are all WHO 3 while hCG is elevated and emergency contraception (EC) is also permitted (WHO 3) – see UKMEC.
  - Combined hormonal methods can be used as soon as hCG concentrations are normal.
  - Intrauterine methods are *not* recommended (WHO 4) until a normal menstrual cycle is established.
  - If frank cancer is diagnosed, with chemotherapy in progress, take advice from the regional centre: a progestogen-only method such as Cerazette would often be best.

The important point is that, after the all-clear with respect to hCG monitoring has been given by the regional centre, this past history becomes irrelevant: and any hormonal or intrauterine method is usable (WHO 1).

Carcinomas of the ovary and of the endometrium

The good news is that both are definitely less frequent in COC-users. Numerous studies have shown that the incidence of both is roughly halved among all users, and reduced to one-third in long-term users; a protective effect can be detected in ex-users for up to 10–15 years. Suppression of ovulation in COC-users and of normal mitotic activity in the endometrium are the accepted explanations of these findings.

> **Clinical implications**
> It would be reasonable for a woman known to be predisposed to either of these cancers to choose to use the COC primarily for this protective effect.

Colorectal cancer

There are suggestive data, though the case is not yet fully proven, that the Pill may also *protect* against this cancer.

Other cancers

Associations have been mooted but not confirmed.

> **Clinically**
> Women who are apparently cured by local radical surgery for neoplasia of the ovary, cervix and uterus and for malignant melanoma may all use COCs.

Benefits and risks – a summary

The 'bottom line' when counselling COC-takers is as follows: *Populations using the Pill may develop different benign or malignant neoplasms from control populations, but it does not appear from computer modelling studies that the overall risk of neoplasia is increased. See Figure 4.*

Circulatory disease and choice of COC

Venous thromboembolism

A massive UK 'Pill-scare' in 1995 could have been minimized if the data had been presented as a *reduction* in risk of venous thromboembolism (VTE) for women using levonorgestrel (LNG)

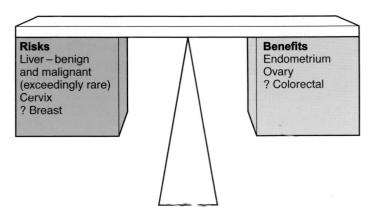

Figure 4
Cancer and COCs: a balance.

or norethisterone (NET) pills. This would have been presentationally better, explaining to the public and the media that 'the bottle is half full – not half empty!' But it would also have been scientifically more valid, as that is where the difference lies: the *different* progestogens are really LNG and to a lesser extent NET, not the 'third-generation' progestogens desogestrel (DSG) and gestodene (GSD), which were adversely highlighted at the time.

LNG has been shown to oppose any estrogen-mediated rise in sex-hormone-binding globulin (SHBG) and in high-density lipoprotein (HDL) cholesterol – and can even lower the latter if enough is given. See Figure 5. Somatically, it also opposes the tendency for estrogen to improve acne. It is thus unlike most other marketed progestogens, which basically allow estrogen to 'do its own thing' in a dose-dependent way. Researchers in the Netherlands and the UK have now shown that LNG when combined with EE reduces the procoagulant effects of the latter on acquired activated protein C resistance and the reduction of protein S levels. Hence it is no longer biologically implausible that the combination of LNG with EE would reduce the clinical risk of venous thrombosis to below what it would be with a given dose of EE alone. It looks as though DSG and GSD, and indeed most probably the other progestogens used for contraception,

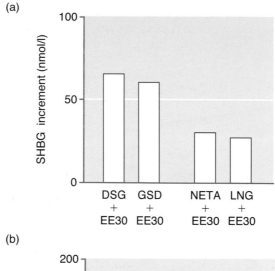

(a)

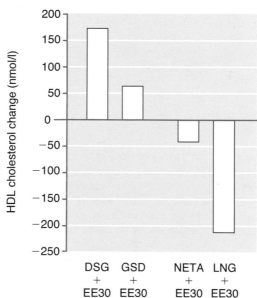

(b)

Figure 5
Prospective randomized controlled trials of four pills: desogestrel (DSG) + ethinylestradiol (EE) 30; gestodene (GSD) + EE30; norethisterone acetate (NETA) + EE30; levonorgestrel (LNG) + EE30. (a) Increment in sex-hormone-binding globulin (SHBG). (b) Change in high-density lipoprotein (HDL) cholesterol. (Margaret Pyke Centre Study.)

simply fail to have that opposing action – just as they do when we actually want a greater estrogenic effect (e.g. when choosing a Pill for someone with acne, for which it is well known that LNG products are less good).

Norgestimate (NGM), the progestogen used in Cilest and Evra, the contraceptive patch, is in part metabolized to LNG. Yet both these two combination products with EE are more estrogen-dominant than Microgynon 30.

Any beneficial effect of LNG (and NET and its pro-drugs) on VTE risk may not be as great as the epidemiology of 1995–96 suggested. This is because of the influence of prescriber bias, the 'healthy-user' effect and so-called 'attrition of the susceptibles' – which led, at the time of the studies, to:

- women at lower intrinsic risk being more likely to be left using the older LNG or NET Pills – because the women with risk factors such as smoking and high body mass index (BMI) had been switched to what were thought to be the 'safer' newer products with which they were compared! Hence (the mirror image):
- women at higher intrinsic risk tending to be users of DSG and GSD products.

Clinical implications

Advice from the UK Department of Health (DoH), issued after the 1998 review by the Medicines Commission of the VTE issue still provides a good bottom-line with regard to the COC and this one condition. They 'found no new safety concerns' about third-generation DSG or GSD products, and went on:

The spontaneous incidence of VTE in healthy non-pregnant women (not taking any oral contraceptive) is about 5 cases per 100 000 women per year. The incidence in users of second generation Pills is about 15 per 100 000 women per year of use. The incidence in users of third generation Pills is about 25 cases per 100 000 women per year of use: this excess incidence has not been satisfactorily explained by bias or confounding. The level of all of these risks of VTE increases with age and is likely to be increased in women with other known risk factors for VTE such as obesity.

> 'Women must be fully informed of these very small risks . . .
> Provided they are, the type of Pill is for the woman together with
> her doctor or other family planning professionals jointly to decide
> in the light of her individual medical history.' [Author's emphasis.]
> DoH 7 April 1979

The above absolute rates of VTE are still disputed by some authorities, and by the manufacturers of DSG and GSD products. Even if the whole difference is accepted as real, Table 4 and Figure 6, where the denominator is per million rather than per 100 000, help to put the risks into perspective:

- Using the incidence rates given by the DoH above, each year there will be 100 fewer cases of VTE per million users of an LNG product such as Microgynon 30 (Schering Health Care) than

Table 4
Comparative risks[a]

Annual risks per 1 000 000 women		
Activity	**Cases**	**Deaths**
Having a baby, UK (all direct causes of death)		60
Having a baby (VTE)[b]	600	20
Using DSG/GSD pill (VTE)[b]	250	5
Using LNG/NET pill (VTE)[b]	150	3
Non-user, non-pregnant (VTE)[b]	50–100	1–2
Risk from *all causes* through COC (healthy non-smoking woman)		10
Home accidents		30
Playing soccer		40
Road accidents		80
Parachuting (10 jumps/year)		200
Scuba diving		220
Hang-gliding		1500
Cigarette smoking (in next year if aged 35)		1670
Death from pregnancy/ childbirth in rural Africa		≥10 000

[a]Sources: Dinman BD. *JAMA* 1980; **244**: 1226–8; Mills A et al. *BMJ* 1996; **312**: 121; Anon. *BMJ* 1991; **302**: 743; Strom B. *Pharmacoepidemiology*, 2nd edn. Chichester: Wiley, 1994: 57–65; www.doh.gov.uk/cmo/mdeaths.htm.

[b]VTE rates are for idiopathic cases, with no other risk factor; VTE mortality rate is assumed to be 2%, but to be higher for VTE occurring in pregnancy.

among a similar number of women using a more estrogen-dominant product. Using an estimate of 2% for VTE mortality in the UK, this means a 2 per million greater annual VTE mortality for such a product than say Microgynon 30. From Figure 6, this risk difference is the same as that from 2 hours of driving.

- Hence, if a woman chooses (as she might very reasonably do, after counselling), to control a symptom such as acne by switching away from Microgynon 30 to an estrogen-dominant product: all she needs to do is avoid one 2-hour drive in the whole of the next year to remain, in terms of VTE risk, effectively still on the Microgynon 30!
- The risk difference is tiny but probably real – and therefore worth avoiding by the current UK policy of generally using a LNG product as first line, while being fully prepared to switch for symptom control upon request.
- The primary reason for choosing, or changing to, a more estrogenic product, such as one containing DSG or GSD as the progestogen, is for the control of side effects occurring on a LNG or NET product.

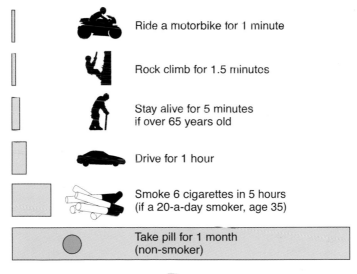

Figure 6
Time required to have a 1:1 000 000 risk of dying. (Adapted from Minerva, British Medical Journal, 1988.)

Arterial diseases: acute myocardial infarction, haemorrhagic stroke and ischaemic stroke

Epidemiology, spearheaded by the WHO, has shown that the COC was not the prime cause of most of the arterial events occurring in Pill-takers, both within and outside research studies. The COC was blamed, yet arterial disease is exceptionally rare in COC-takers during the reproductive years, aside from an increasing risk with *age,* unless they also *smoke* or have *diabetes or hypertension. Migraine* is a specific, independent risk factor for ischaemic stroke.

- **Acute myocardial infarction (AMI)**. The odds ratio (OR) of this condition in some studies goes up from unity (no added risk) in non-smoking controls, to 10 or more in smokers also taking the COC: who indeed are in double jeopardy, since the case-fatality rate of AMI when it occurs in smokers who use the COC is also much higher.
- **Haemorrhagic stroke (HS), including subarachnoid haemorrhage**. The WHO and other studies have failed to show any increased risk due to the COC under age 35 unless there is also a risk factor such as hypertension (OR 10) or smoking (OR 3). The risk increases with age, and this effect is magnified by current COC use, but with no effect of past use or long-duration use.
- **Ischaemic stroke (IS).** Here, even in non-smokers, there is a detectable increase in the OR due to pill-taking in the range of 1.5 to a maximum of 2. Much of this risk seems to be focused within the subpopulation who suffer from migraine with aura (see below). The OR for hypertension is 3, as is that for smoking 3.
- **Effect of dose/type of hormone.** It is believed, though never proven, that the modern low-estrogen pills help to minimize the arterial risks, as has been shown (at least for the comparison between doses less than and more than 50 μg) for VTE. Whether the type of progestogen in the COC separately affects (as it can only do in those with risk factors) the above arterial conditions is still uncertain.

Prescribing guidelines

Current scientific evidence suggests only two prerequisites for the safe provision of COCs: a careful personal and family history with particular attention to cardiovascular risk factors, and a well-taken blood pressure [Hannaford P, Webb A. Evidence-guided prescribing of combined oral contraceptives: consensus statement. *Contraception* 1996; **54**: 125–9]. To this should be added, crucially, measurement of the woman's BMI at presentation.

- Prescribers should always take a comprehensive personal and family history to exclude **absolute and relative contraindications** to the use of COCs (see pp. 33–38).
- A personal history of definite VTE remains an absolute contraindication to any hormonal method containing EE (including Evra or NuvaRing), combined with any progestogen.
- The risk factors for risk of future VTE and arterial wall disease must be assessed (see Tables 5 and 6).
- Note that it now appears, after years of uncertainty in the literature, that smoking is an independent risk factor for VTE, as well as arterial disease.
- Alone, one risk factor from either Table 5 or 6 is a relative contraindication (WHO 2 or 3 columns), unless it is particularly severe (WHO 4 column).
- Synergism means that if WHO 3 already applies, any additional risk factor moves the category to WHO 4 ('Do not use').
- Generally, however, COC use is acceptable on a WHO 3 basis when two WHO 2 factors apply.

The remarks and footnotes in Tables 5 and 6 are fundamental to Pill prescribing.

Hereditary predispositions to VTE (thrombophilias)

Almost the only indication for screening is a strong family history of one or more siblings or parents having had a spontaneous VTE under the age of 45. This justifies testing for the genetic predispositions, including factor V Leiden (the genetic cause of activated protein C resistance), which if identified is classified as WHO 4. Even if all the results are normal, however, the COC remains WHO 2. The woman's strong family history cannot be discounted, since by no means all the predisposing abnormalities of the complex haemostatic system have yet been characterized. This is why blanket screening by any blood test is not justifiable – the cost would be prohibitive and, in terms of what matters, which is the occurrence of actual disease events, there are just too many false negatives and positives.

Table 5
Risk factors for venous thromboembolism (VTE).

Risk factor	Absolute contraindication WHO 4	Relative contraindication WHO 3	WHO 2	Remarks
Personal or family history (FH) of thrombophilias, *or* of venous thrombosis in sibling or parent	Past VTE event; or identified clotting abnormality in this person, whether hereditary or acquired FH of a defined thrombophilia *or* *idiopathic* thrombotic event in parent or sibling <45 and thrombophilia screen not (yet) available	FH of thrombosis in parent or sibling <45 with recognized precipitating factor (e.g. major surgery, postpartum) and thrombophilia screen not available	FH of thrombotic event in parent or sibling <45 with or without a recognized precipitating factor and *Normal* thrombophilia screen FH in parent or sibling ≥45 or FH in 2nd-degree relative (classified WHO 2 but tests not indicated)	*Idiopathic* VTE in a parent or sibling <45 is an indication for a thrombophilia screen if available. The decision to undertake screening in other situations (including where there was a recognized precipitating factor), will be unusual because very cost-ineffective – might be done on clinical grounds, in discussion with the woman Even a normal thrombophilia screen cannot be entirely reassuring, as some predispositions not yet known
Overweight (high BMI)	BMI >39	BMI 30–39	BMI 25–29	

Risk factor				
Immobility	Bed-bound, with or without major surgery; or leg fractured and immobilized	Wheelchair life, debilitating illness	Reduced mobility for other reason	
Varicose veins (VVs)	Current superficial vein thrombosis in the upper thigh. Current sclerotherapy for VVs (until all pressure dressings and bandages removed)		History of superficial vein thrombosis (SVT) in the lower limbs, no deep vein thrombosis	SVT does not result in pulmonary embolism, although this past history means some caution (WHO 2) in case it might be a marker of future VTE risk. Uncomplicated VVs are irrelevant to VTE risk (WHO 1)
Cigarette smoking		≥15 cigarettes per day	<15 cigarettes per day	On balance the literature suggests a VTE risk from smoking, though less than the arterial disease risk it causes
Age >35	>51	35–51, if ex-smoker	35–51 if age is sole risk factor	

Notes

1. A single risk factor in the relative contraindication columns indicates use of LNG/NET pill, if any COC used (as in BNF).
2. Beware of synergism: more than one factor in either of relative contraindication columns. As a working rule, two WHO 2 conditions makes WHO 3; and if WHO 3 applies (e.g. BMI 30–39) addition of either a WHO 3 or WHO 2 (e.g. reduced mobility) condition normally means WHO 4 (do not use).
3. Acquired (non-hereditary) include positive results for anti-phospholipid antibodies – definitely WHO 4 since they also increase the risk of arterial events (Table 6).
4. There are also important acute VTE risk factors, which need to be considered in individual cases: notably major surgery, all leg surgery, long-haul flights and dehydration through any cause.
5. There are minor differences in the above table from UKMEC, notably the author's more cautious categorization of BMIs above 25.

Table 6
Risk factors for arterial disease.

Risk factor	Absolute contraindication WHO 4	Relative contraindication WHO 3	Relative contraindication WHO 2	Remarks
Family history (FH) of atherogenic lipid disorder *or* of arterial CVS event in sibling or parent	Identified familial hyperlipidaemia in this person, persisting despite treatment	FH of known familial lipid disorder or *idiopathic* arterial event in parent or sibling <45 and client's lipid screening result: • not available or • confirmed and responding to treatment	Client has a less problematic common hyperlipidaemia and responding well to treatment FH of arterial event with risk factor (e.g. smoking) in parent or sibling <45 and lipid screen not available	FH of premature (<45) arterial CVS disease without other risk factors, or a known atherogenic lipid disorder in a parent or sibling, indicate fasting lipid screen, if available. (Check with laboratory re clinical implication of abnormal results) Despite any FH, normal lipid screen in client *is* reassuring, and means WHO 1 (in contrast to thrombophilia screening)
Cigarette smoking	≥40 cigarettes/day	15–39 cigarettes/day	<15 cigarettes/day	Cut-offs here are somewhat arbitrary
Diabetes mellitus (DM)	Severe, longstanding DM or end-organ damage (e.g. retinopathy, renal damage, arterial disease)	Not severe/labile and no complications, young patient with short duration of DM		DM is always at least WHO 3 (safer options available)

(condition)				
Hypertension (consistently elevated BP, with appropriate cuff-size and properly taken measurements)	Systolic BP ≥160 mmHg Diastolic BP ≥95 mmHg	Systolic BP in range >140 to 159 mmHg Diastolic BP >90 to 95 mmHg On treatment for essential hypertension, with good control	BP regularly at upper limit of normal (i.e. near to 140/90) Past history of pre-eclampsia (WHO 3 if also a smoker)	Levels for WHO 4 and WHO 3 are consistent with UKMEC
Overweight, high BMI	BMI ≥40	BMI 30–39	BMI 25–29	High BMI increases arterial as well as VTE risk
Migraine	Migraine with aura Migraine without aura if attacks last >72 hours + no overuse of medication	Migraine without aura plus a strong added arterial risk factor	Migraine without aura	Relates to *thrombotic* stroke risk Triptan treatment does not affect the category
Age >35	Age >51 (safer options available)	35–51, if ex-smoker	Age 35–51 if no other risk factors	In persistent smokers, age >35 remains best classified as WHO 4 In ex-smokers, category WHO 3 is because earlier arterial wall damage may persist and safer options available

Notes
1. Beware of synergism: more than one factor in either of relative contraindication columns. As a working rule, two WHO 2 conditions makes WHO 3; and if WHO 3 applies (e.g. smoking ≥15 per day), addition of either a WHO 3 or WHO 2 condition (e.g. age above 35) normally means WHO 4 (as in table).
2. The pill seems to have a negligible, though not nil, adverse effect in arterial disease unless there is a risk factor. In continuing smokers, COC is generally stopped at age 35 in the UK.
3. WHO numbers also relate to use for contraception: use of COCs for medical indications such as PCOS often entails a different risk/benefit analysis, i.e. the extra therapeutic benefits may outweigh expected extra risks.
4. Note: There are minor differences here from UKMEC, notably the author's more cautious categorization with respect to smoking, hyperlipidaemia and DM.

Acquired predispositions to VTE (thrombophilias)

Antiphospholipid antibodies, which increase both VTE and arterial disease risk (Table 6: Note 4) may appear in a number of connective tissue disorders, including systemic lupus erythematosus (SLE). If identified, they absolutely contraindicate COC use (WHO 4).

Which Pills are the current 'best buys' for women?

- **First, all marketed pills are 'in the frame' for prescribing.** Given the tiny possible difference in VTE mortality between the two 'generations', the woman's own choice (initially or at any later stage) of a DSG or GSD or other estrogen-dominant product rather than a LNG or NET one after (well-documented) discussion must be respected. 'The informed user should be the chooser'.
- **First-time users**. Despite what has just been said, it is generally agreed that a low-dose LNG or NET product should remain the *usual* first choice. This is in part because first-timers will include an unknown subgroup who are VTE predisposed, VTE being a more relevant consideration than arterial disease at this age, and the pills suit the majority and cost less. (Consider also offering the use of an ED pill type, to aid in remembering to restart after the pill-free time – see below).
- **In the presence of a single WHO 2 or 3 risk factor for venous thrombosis.** The Summary of Product Characteristics (SPCs) for COCs state that DSG/GSD products are contraindicated.
  - This policy has merit if the COC is to be used *solely for contraception.*
  - However, if there is a clear *therapeutic indication* for the COC, such as the polycystic ovarian syndrome (PCOS) with moderately severe acne, a different risk–benefit balance may apply. Extra therapeutic benefits from a more estrogenic product may be judged to outweigh any expected extra risks (on a WHO 3 basis) because, for example, the woman has a BMI of 32. Relevant choices might be Marvelon 30, Yasmin or Dianette. These probably all share the same (estrogen-dominant) category – but only because they *lack* LNG, with its antagonizing EE effect.
- **Women with a single definite arterial risk factor (Table 6) (e.g. smokers or diabetics) – after a number of**

years VTE-free use or if the COC is used at all by healthy women above the age of 35. As we have seen, in premenopausal women, AMI is almost exclusively a disease of *smokers*. But the hazard is higher when such risk factors are present (the RCGP's relative risk estimate for AMI was 20.8 for smoking Pill-takers!), it increases with age, and the case fatality rate for AMI in Pill-takers is also higher. There is some suggestive evidence that DSG/GSD Pills might have relative advantages for arterial wall disease. Therefore for such *higher-risk women*, or older women aged 35 to 50/51 (provided they are otherwise arterial risk-free), using a 20 μg DSG or GSD product might be (at least) discussed. Any advantages in so doing are far from established, and changing to a different method altogether would usually be a better course. In the UK, Femodette (Schering) (GSD) or Mercilon (Organon) (DSG) are the relevant 20 μg EE products. Loestrin 20 (Galen) would also be acceptable – and preferable if there were any WHO 3-level concern about VTE risk – since it contains a NET-group progestogen.

- **Finally, the primary reason for ever changing COC brands is the control of side effects, for the woman's quality of life.** If, for any indication, she moves to using a product *not* containing LNG or NET, it should be documented that she accepts a possible tiny increase in the risk of VTE. This can be explained as 'in the ballpark' of the risk of driving for 2 hours in the next year (see p. 25).

Eligibility criteria for COCs

Absolute contraindications to COCs or other combined methods (e.g. Evra)

As already mentioned, the contraindications listed below (and in similar subsequent lists of absolute or relative contraindications) are based on WHOMEC, categorised according to the present author's judgement of the evidence – bearing in mind that the WHO has not as yet given its verdict on many issues.

All conditions in this first list are WHO 4 for the COC. However, as will be shown later, for the same conditions progestogen-only pills (POPs), including Cerazette, and other progestogen-only methods, are in most cases classified no higher than WHO 2.

1. Past or present circulatory disease

- Any past proven arterial or venous thrombosis
- Ischaemic heart disease or angina or coronary arteritis (Kawasaki disease – past history is WHO 3 or 2, depending on completeness of recovery)
- Severe or combined risk factors for venous or arterial disease (see Tables 5 and 6) can be WHO 4 – e.g. BMI 40 or above is sufficient on its own for the WHO 4 category
- Atherogenic lipid disorders (take advice from an expert)
- Known prothrombotic states:
  - abnormality of coagulation/fibrinolysis, i.e. any of above congenital or acquired thrombophilia states
  - from at least 2 (preferably 4) weeks before until 2 weeks after mobilization following elective major or leg surgery (do not demand that the COC be stopped for minor surgery such as laparoscopy)
  - during leg immobilization (e.g. after fracture) or varicose vein injection treatment
  - when going to high altitudes if there are added risk factors (otherwise WHO 3 – see below)
- Migraine with aura (described on pp. 39–40)
- Definite aura *without* following a headache
- Transient ischaemic attacks
- Past cerebral haemorrhage
- Pulmonary hypertension, any cause
- Structural (uncorrected) heart disease such as valvular heart disease or shunts/septal defects is only WHO 4 if there is an added arterial or venous thromboembolic risk (persisting, if there has been surgery). Always discuss this with the cardiologist – could be WHO 3, especially if the patient is always on warfarin. Important WHO 4 examples are:
  - atrial fibrillation or flutter whether sustained or paroxysmal – or not current but high risk (e.g. mitral stenosis)
  - dilated left atrium (>4 cm)
  - cyanotic heart disease
  - any dilated cardiomyopathy; but this is classified as only WHO 2 with a *past* history of any type (including pregnancy cardiomyopathy), when in full remission
- In other structural heart conditions, if there is little or no direct or indirect risk of thromboembolism (this being the crucial point to check with the cardiologist), the COC is usable (WHO 3 or 2)

2. Liver

- Active liver cell disease (whenever liver function tests are currently abnormal, including infiltrations, severe chronic hepatitis B and C, and cirrhosis)
- Past Pill-related cholestatic jaundice; if this was in pregnancy, it

can be WHO 3 (contrast WHOMEC and UKMEC, who say WHO 3 not 4 for the former – and WHO 2 for the latter)
- Dubin–Johnson and Rotor syndromes (Gilbert's disease is WHO 2)
- Following viral hepatitis or other liver cell damage: but COCs may be resumed once liver function tests have become normal and a dose of ≤2 units of alcohol consumption is tolerated
- Liver adenoma, carcinoma
- Acute hepatic porphyrias; other porphyrias are usually WHO 3, but a non-steroid hormone method is usually preferable

3. History of serious condition affected by sex steroids or related to previous COC use
- SLE – also a VTE risk
- COC-induced hypertension
- Pancreatitis due to hypertriglyceridaemia
- Pemphigoid gestationis
- Chorea
- Stevens–Johnson syndrome (erythema multiforme), if COC-associated
- Trophoblastic disease – but only until hCG levels are undetectable
- Haemolytic uraemic syndrome (HUS) and thrombotic thrombocytopenic purpura (TTP); HUS in the past may sometimes be WHO 3 (see below)

4. Pregnancy

5. Undiagnosed genital tract bleeding

6. Estrogen-dependent neoplasms
- Breast cancer
- Past breast biopsy showing premalignant epithelial atypia

7. Miscellaneous
- Allergy to any Pill constituent
- Past benign intracranial hypertension
- Specific to Yasmin: because of the unique spironolactone-like effects of the contained progestogen drospirenone, this particular brand should be avoided – should a COC be appropriate – in anyone at risk of high potassium levels (including severe renal insufficiency, hepatic dysfunction and treatment with potassium-sparing diuretics)
- Sturge–Weber syndrome (thrombotic stroke risk)
- Post-partum for 6 weeks if breastfeeding (according to UKMEC)

8. Woman's anxiety about COC safety unrelieved by counselling

Note that several of the above (e.g. 4, 5 and 8) are not necessarily permanent contraindications. Moreover, many women over the years have been unnecessarily deprived of COCs for reasons now shown to have no link, such as thrush; or that would have positively benefited from the method, such as secondary amenorrhoea with hypo-estrogenism.

Relative contraindications to combined oral contraceptives (COCs)

Below are listed the *relative* contraindications to COCs, WHO 2 or 3, signifying that the COC method is usable in context with:

- the benefit–risk evaluation for that individual
- the acceptability or otherwise of alternatives
- sometimes with special advice (e.g. in migraine, to report a change of symptomatology) or monitoring.

In cases with excess risk of venous thrombosis (e.g. wheelchair life – WHO 3 – see Table 5), if the Pill is used at all for contraception, it should be a LNG/NET variety.

Relative contraindications to COCs are WHO 2, here, unless otherwise stated:
- Risk factors for arterial or venous disease (see Tables 5 and 6). These are WHO 2, sometimes 3 (e.g. in my view any BMI above 30 is at least WHO 3): provided that only one is present and that not of such severity as to justify WHO 4 (e.g. BMI 40+)
  - HUS (see above): in past history may be WHO 3 if complete recovery and not Pill-associated (e.g. past *Escherichia coli* O157 infection as established cause of past attack of HUS)
  - Diabetes (minimum category being WHO 3), hypertensive disease and migraine all deserve separate discussion (see below)
  - Postpartum during the first 3 weeks (WHO 3 due to postdelivery VTE risk, but negligible fertility anyway).
- Risk of altitude illness is not more probable because a climber is on COC; but if it occurs, in its most severe forms venous or arterial thromboembolism or patchy pulmonary hypertension are known to occur, any of which would contraindicate the method. Hence all women travelling to above 2500 m should be informed that the COC might increase the thrombotic component of severe arterial illness if that were to occur. The COC would be WHO 3, in general, but could be only WHO 2 in many healthy trekkers who intend always to follow the maxim 'climb high but sleep low'. More details are given in *BMJ* 2003; **326**: 915–19.

- Sex-steroid-dependent cancer in prolonged remission (WHO 3) – prolonged is defined as after 5 years by WHOMEC: prime example is breast cancer.
- Malignant melanoma is not related so WHO 2 for the Pill.
- If a young (<40 years of age) first-degree relative has breast cancer or the woman herself has benign breast disease (UKMEC says WHO 1). Being a known carrier of one of the BRCA genes is WHO 3 (p. 17).
- During the monitoring of abnormal cervical smears (WHO 2).
- During and after definitive treatment for CIN (WHO 2).
- Oligo/amenorrhoea (COCs may be prescribed, after investigation – may be WHO 1, use unrestricted, if the purpose is to supply estrogen in a woman needing contraception or to control the symptoms of PCOS).
- Hyperprolactinaemia (WHO 3, but only for patients who are on specialist drug treatment and with close supervision).
- Most chronic congenital or acquired syctemic diseases (see below) are WHO 2.
- Sickle cell trait is WHO 1, but homozygous sickle cell disease is WHO 2 (although DMPA is preferred for this).
- Inflammatory bowel disease is WHO 2, or (my view) WHO 3 if severe, because of VTE risk in exacerbations.
- Otosclerosis (WHO 2).
- Gallstones (WHO 3, but WHO 2 after cholecystectomy).
- Very severe depression, if there is a clear history of it being exacerbated by COCs (but unwanted pregnancies can be very depressing!).
- Diseases that require long-term treatment with enzyme-inducing drugs are WHO 3 (COC is usable – see below – but alternative contraception is preferred).

Intercurrent diseases

It is impossible for the lists above to include every known disease that might have a bearing (i.e. WHO 4, 3 or 2) on COC prescription, and for many the data are unavailable. A working protocol is therefore:

- First, ascertain whether or not the condition might lead to **summation** with known major adverse effects of COCs, particularly thrombotic risk. If so, this usually means WHO 4, sometimes 3.
- If there are no grounds to expect summation of risk, in most serious chronic conditions the patient can be reassured that

COCs are not known to have any effect – good or bad. They may then be used (WHO 2), though with careful monitoring and alertness for the onset of new risk factors.
- The reliable protection from pregnancy that the COC can offer is often particularly important when other diseases are present, although we do now have other reliable choices that are free of EE and therefore of thrombotic risk (e.g. Cerazette, Implanon, IUDs and the IUS).

Diabetes mellitus

In general, and whether of Type 1 or Type 2, in the present author's view, this is a WHO 3 condition even when there is no *known* diabetic tissue damage (cf. WHOMEC, which classes well-controlled diabetes mellitus (DM) as WHO 2).

Clinically, given the high arterial disease risk, in particular, the POP (often Cerazette) or Implanon are definitely preferred alternatives. These can be started following coitarche in the young; with perhaps a modern copper IUD, the LNG-IUS or sterilization to follow, as appropriate.

Mercilon, Femodette or Loestrin 20 (see above) are COC options – but for limited duration and under careful supervision: for cases where there is no known arteriopathy, retinopathy, neuropathy or renal damage, nor any added arterial risk factor such as obesity or smoking – all of which mean WHO 4 – and preferably if the duration of the disease has been short (Table 6).

Hypertension

Hypertension is an important risk factor for both heart disease and stroke (see Table 6).

- In most women on COCs, there is a slight increase in both systolic and diastolic BP within the normotensive range: less than 1% become clinically hypertensive with modern low doses, but the rate increases with age and duration of use. Above 140/90 mmHg, this is classified as WHO 3; but if BP is repeatedly above 160/95 (either the systolic or diastolic figure. I agree here with UKMEC, whose trigger for action is more cautious than WHOMEC), the method should be stopped; and even if it then normalizes, this Pill-induced hypertension means WHO 4 for the future.

> - Past severe toxaemia (pregnancy-induced hypertension) does not predispose to hypertension during COC use, but it is a risk factor for myocardial infarction (WHO 2) – markedly so if the women also smokes (WHO 3).
> - Essential hypertension (not COC-related), when well controlled on drugs, is WHO 3: i.e. the COC is usable, but not preferred.

Migraine

Like hypertension, this condition is of critical relevance both at the first prescription and during the follow-up of COC-takers.

> **Migraines can be defined by the answers to the following questions:**
> *'During the last 3 months did you have the following with your headaches?*
> 1. You felt **nauseated** or sick in your stomach?
> 2. You were **bothered by light** a lot more than when you don't have headache.
> 3. Your headaches **limited your ability** to work, study or do what you needed to do for at least 1 day.'
>
> Two 'yes' answers out of the three means a diagnosis of migraine.

Migraine and stroke risk

- Studies have shown an increased risk of ischaemic stroke in migraine sufferers and in COC-users, and if combined, there is 'summation' of risk.
- There is good evidence of exacerbation of risk by arterial risk factors, including smoking and increasing age above 35 years.
- The presence of aura *before* (or sometimes even without) the headache is the main marker of risk (WHO 4) – indeed, not only for ischaemic stroke but also for coronary artery disease and myocardial infarction. But it seems increasingly likely that there is no significantly increased risk through having migraine without aura – though for the present this is still classified as WHO 2. Given that the 1-year prevalence of any migraine in women has been shown to be as high as 18%, it is crucial to identify the important subgroup with aura (1-year prevalence about 5%).

Migraine with aura

- Taking this crucial history starts by establishing the timing: *neurological symptoms of aura begin before the headache itself*, and typically last around 20–30 minutes (maximum 60 minutes) and stop before the headache (which may be very mild). Headache may start as aura is resolving, or there may be a gap of up to 1 hour.

- Visual symptoms occur in 99% of true auras, and hence should be asked about first.
- These are typically bright and affect part of the *field* of vision, on the same side in both eyes (homonymous hemianopia).
- Fortification spectra are often described, typically a bright scintillating zig-zag line gradually enlarging from a bright centre on one side, to form a convex C-shape surrounding the area of lost vision (which is a *bright* scotoma).
- Sensory symptoms are confirmatory of aura, occurring in around one third of cases and rarely in the absence of visual aura. Typically, they come as 'pins and needles' (paraesthesia) spreading up one arm or one side of the face or the tongue; the leg is rarely affected. They are positive symptoms – *not loss* of function.
- Disturbance of speech may also occur, in the form of nominal dysphasia.

Note the absence in the above list of the symptoms that occur during headache itself (photophobia or *generalised* blurring or 'flashing lights'). Moreover, aura symptoms should not be confused with *premonitory symptoms*, such as food cravings, excessive lethargy, extra sensitivity to light and sound, occurring a day or so before any migraine (i.e. with or without aura) and continuing into the headache.

Clinical implications

- Ask the woman to describe a typical attack from the very beginning, including any symptoms before a headache. Listen to what she says, *but at the same time watch her carefully*.
- A most useful **sign** that what she describes is likely to be true aura is if *she waves her hand on one or other side of her own head and draws something like a zig-zag line in the air*.

In summary, aura has three main features:
- Characteristic **timing**: Onset *before* (headache) + duration up to 1 hour + resolution before or with onset of headache
- Symptoms **visual** (99%)
- Description **visible** (using a hand).

Migraine-related absolute contraindications (WHO 4) to starting or continuing the COC

- *Migraine with aura* or *aura without headache*. The *artificial estrogen* of the COC is what needs to be avoided (or stopped, at once and forever) to minimize the additional risk of a thrombotic stroke.
- *Other migraines (even without aura) that are exceptionally severe in a COC-taker* and last more than 72 hours despite optimal medication.
- *All migraines treated with ergot derivatives*, due to their vasoconstrictor actions.
- *Migraine without aura* **plus** multiple risk factors for arterial disease, or a relevant interacting disease (e.g. connective tissue diseases already linked with stroke risk), and according to UKMEC above age 35 the COC should be discontinued in *all* migraine sufferers (WHO 4).

Note that in all of the above circumstances, any of the *progesto-gen-only* (i.e. *estrogen-free*) hormonal methods may be offered immediately. Similar headaches may continue, but now without the potential added risk from prothrombotic effects of EE. Particularly useful choices are the POP (Cerazette in the young), Implanon, the LNG-IUS, or a modern copper IUD (all WHO 1 in my view, although strangely WHOMEC and UKMEC both classify the first three as WHO 2 or even 3).

Migraine: relative contraindications for the COC

WHO 2. The COC is 'broadly usable' in the following cases:
- *Migraine without aura*, and also without any arterial risk factor from Table 6 and still under the age of 35. Note that if these (or indeed other 'ordinary' headaches) occur only or mainly in the pill-free interval (PFI), tricycling the COC may help.
- *Use of a triptan drug* in the absence of any other contraindicating factors.
- *The occurrence of a woman's first-ever attack of migraine without aura while on the COC*. It is a reasonable precaution to stop the Pill if she is seen during the attack. But after full evaluation of the symptoms – provided there were no features of aura or marked risk factors – the COC can be later restarted (WHO 2), with the usual counselling/caveats about future aura.

WHO 3. The COC is usable with caution and close supervision:

- *Primarily*, this means migraine without aura (common/simple migraine) where there is also an important risk factor for ischaemic stroke present. A good example is heavy smoking, which itself is a significant risk factor of ischaemic stroke.
- *Secondly*, a clear past history of typical migraine *with aura* more than 5 years earlier or only during pregnancy, with no recurrence, may be regarded as WHO 3. COCs may be given a trial, with counselling and regular supervision, along with a specific warning that the onset of definite aura (carefully explained) means that the user should:
  - stop the Pill immediately
  - use alternative contraception, and
  - seek medical advice as soon as possible.

Differential diagnoses

It may be difficult to distinguish such relatively common, migraine-associated transient ischaemia from rare organic episodes – true transient ischaemic attacks (TIAs) (e.g. due to paradoxical embolism, which is an established risk of an atrial septal defect or persistent foramen ovale). TIAs are more sudden in onset than migraine aura and last over an hour, without other migraine symptoms such as nausea.

Upon suspicion these of course mean the same in practice, i.e. WHO 4 – *stop the pill immediately*. If an organic episode is a possibility, hospital investigation should also follow.

The following features are not typical of migraine

- focal epilepsy, severe acute vertigo, hemiparesis, ataxia, aphasia or unilateral tinnitus
- a severe unexplained drop attack or collapse
- monocular blindness (black scotoma) – this could rarely be a retinal vascular event or a symptom of TIA (amaurosis fugax)
- progressive or persistent neurological symptoms (migraine is episodic, with complete freedom from symptoms between attacks).

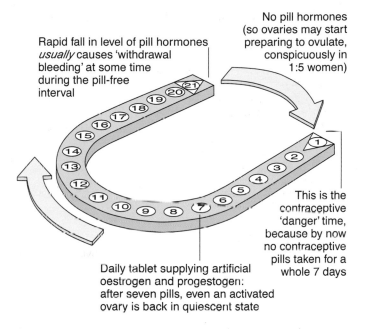

Rapid fall in level of pill hormones *usually* causes 'withdrawal bleeding' at some time during the pill-free interval

No pill hormones (so ovaries may start preparing to ovulate, conspicuously in 1:5 women)

This is the contraceptive 'danger' time, because by now no contraceptive pills taken for a whole 7 days

Daily tablet supplying artificial oestrogen and progestogen: after seven pills, even an activated ovary is back in quiescent state

Figure 7
'Horseshoe' analogy to explain the 21-day cycle. Omission of tablets either side of the gap in the horseshoe lengthens the 'contraception-losing interval'. See text.

The 'pill-free interval' and its implications for COC prescribing and maintenance of efficacy

As no contraceptive is being taken during the PFI, it has important efficacy implications (Figure 7). Biochemical and ultrasound data obtained at the MPC and elsewhere demonstrate return of significant pituitary and ovarian follicular activity during the PFI in about 20% of cases – to a marked extent in some – but even in these cases, renewed pill-taking after no more than a 7-day PFI restores ovarian quiescence. However, these data make it clear that any lengthening of the PFI beyond 7 days is likely to lead to breakthrough ovulation. Lengthening of the PFI might be caused either side of the 'horseshoe' in Figure 7; i.e. from omissions, malabsorption as from vomiting (an advantage of the new non-oral combined products Evra and NuvaRing), or drug interactions that involve pills *either at the start or at the end of a packet*.

All prospective COC-users need warning about this, as their initial thought is bound to be that the 'worst' pills to miss would be in the middle of a packet (i.e. they use the wrong analogy with the middle of a normal cycle). Indeed, a good mantra for all COC pill-takers as they leave their first counselling visit is *'I must never be a "late-restarter"'*.

In 1986, a population of current Pill-users was studied after the end of a routine PFI. The study showed that if only 14 or even as few as 7 pills were then taken, no fertile ovulation occurred after 7 pills were subsequently missed. This and other work may be summarized as follows:

- Seven consecutive pills are enough 'to shut the door' on the ovaries (therefore pills 8–21, or longer during tricycling, simply 'keep the door shut')
- Seven pills can be omitted without ovulation, as indeed is regularly the case in the PFI
- More than seven pills missed (*in total*) risks ovulation.

Clinical implications

On the evidence available, WHO, in the WHOSPR, is now comfortable to define a 'missed pill' as one that is 24 hours late (not 12 hours, as hitherto). But it has unhelpfully proposed *two* protocols based on the above pharmacology: one for up to 20 μg EE-containing products and one for higher doses. UKMEC suggests the same, but there is continuing disagreement between authorities as to the best advice for pill-takers in the UK context.

Given the known marked individual variation in ovarian responses, with greater significance for efficacy in a particular woman than the pill dose she takes, this author favours instructions based on the more cautious of WHO's suggested protocols: giving the same advice regardless of the formulation, based on what WHO recommends for the lowest available COC doses. There are just three points to make:

1. **'ONE tablet missed, for up to 24 hours':** aside from taking the delayed pill and the next one on time, no special action is needed. This applies up to the time that two tablets would need to be taken at once, 'to catch up'. **'ANYTHING MORE THAN ONE tablet missed'** (i.e. a second tablet is also late by one or more hours): Use CONDOMS as well, for the next 7 days

Plus:
2. If this happened in the third active pill-week, at the end of pack RUN ON to the next pack (skipping seven placebos if present)

And:
3. In the first pill week, EMERGENCY CONTRACEPTION is recommended IF, with sexual exposure since the last pack, the COC-user is a '*late restarter*' by more than 2 days (>9-day PFI) or more than two pills are missed (or, she had a >9 day PFI through missed pills at *end of last pack*). This should be followed, next day, by taking the appropriate day's tablet.

As an alternative, Figure 8 presents the same advice in a flowchart.

Note that this removes the emergency contraception recommendation altogether where omissions occur in the second or third week of tablet taking. After all, if a pill-user omits say three pills in the third week and follows instruction 2 above so that she misses her next routine PFI by running on to the next pack, she will be even *less* likely to ovulate than usual. Even if she omits all 7 pills in the second or third week, the 7 or 14 pills she *has* taken will have made her ovary quiescent so, to quote above, 'seven tablets can be missed without ovulation'.

If 28-day packs are used (Microgynon ED, which usefully helps to avoid risky 'late restarts'), the user must learn which are the dummy 'reminder' tablets. If she ever makes her own PFI break prematurely − another way of saying that she has missed some of the last seven active pills − these placebos must be omitted.

After pill-taking errors or severe vomiting or short-term use of an enzyme-inducer drug (see below), all women should be asked to report back if they have no withdrawal bleeding in the *next* PFI.

Every time you miss any one pill (late by up to 24 hours):

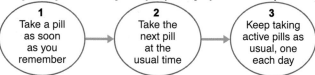

| **1** Take a pill as soon as you remember | → | **2** Take the next pill at the usual time | → | **3** Keep taking active pills as usual, one each day |

If you miss more than 1 pill – meaning anything *more* than 24 hours have elapsed since the time an active pill should have been taken:

4
As well as 1–3, avoid sex or use an extra method for 7 days and:

In these special cases, ALSO follow these special rules:

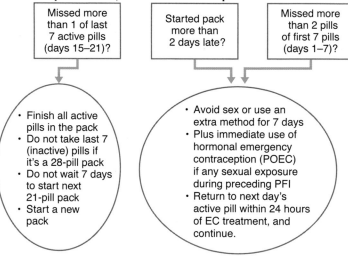

| Missed more than 1 of last 7 active pills (days 15–21)? | Started pack more than 2 days late? | Missed more than 2 pills of first 7 pills (days 1–7)? |

- Finish all active pills in the pack
- Do not take last 7 (inactive) pills if it's a 28-pill pack
- Do not wait 7 days to start next 21-pill pack
- Start a new pack

- Avoid sex or use an extra method for 7 days
- Plus immediate use of hormonal emergency contraception (POEC) if any sexual exposure during preceding PFI
- Return to next day's active pill within 24 hours of EC treatment, and continue.

If you miss any of the 7 inactive pills (in a 28-pill[b] pack only):

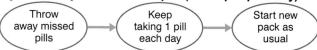

| Throw away missed pills | → | Keep taking 1 pill each day | → | Start new pack as usual |

Figure 8 *Advice for missed pills. (Repill-days 8–14, see p. 45).*
[a]*This can mean taking two pills at once, both when you would normally take the second. (But if it is any later, see the 'more than 1 pill' advice.)*
[b]*28-pill (ED) packs can obviously help some pill-takers not to forget to restart after each PFI (the contraception-losing interval). See p. 45. Even with triphasic pills, you should go straight to (the first phase of) the same brand. You may bleed a bit but you will still strengthen your contraception.*

Vomiting and diarrhoea

If vomiting began over 2 hours after a pill was taken, it can be assumed to have been absorbed. Otherwise follow advice in box on page 45 or Figure 8, according to the number and timing of the tablets deemed to have been missed. Diarrhoea alone is not a problem, unless it is of cholera-like severity.

Previous COC failure

Women who have had a previous COC failure may claim perfect compliance or perhaps admit to omission of no more than one pill. Either way, as surveys show, most women miss a tablet quite frequently yet rarely conceive, so pill failure tells us more about the individual's physiology than her memory. She is likely to be a member of that one-fifth of the population whose ovaries show above-average return to activity in the PFI. Such women (if not now choosing a LARC) may therefore be advised to take either three or four packets in a row (Figure 9) followed by a shortened PFI. Both of these regimens are often termed *tricycling*. The gap is shortened usually to 4 days, in high conception-risk cases – such as this or during the use of enzyme inducers (see below).

Once it has been appreciated that the Achilles' heel of the COC is the PFI, the COC can always be made 'stronger' as a contraceptive, by eliminating and/or shortening the PFI through numerous variations on the tricycling theme depicted in Figure 9 (see also *bicycling*, below).

Why have PFIs at all? Various ways to 'tricycle' the Pill

The pill-free week does promote a reassuring withdrawal bleed (and, indeed, if this does not occur in two successive cycles, it

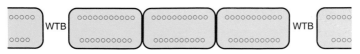

Figure 9
Tricycling (three or four – or more – packs in a row). Note the use of monophasic packs – as in Seasonale which equates to 4 packs in a row. Duration of PFI may also be shortened from 7 to 4 days: see text. WTB, withdrawal bleeds.

is best to eliminate pregnancy using a sensitive urine test). If this bleed is not seen as important, and to obtain certain other advantages in the 'tricycling' box below, any woman may omit most or all the PFIs and associated bleeds as a long-term *option*.

Seasonale is a dedicated tricycle-type packaging in the USA that provides four packets of the formulation of Microgynon (Schering Health Care)/Ovranette (Wyeth Laboratories) in a row, followed by a 7-day pill-free week, such that the user has a bleed every 3 months (i.e. seasonally!). This variant requires 16 packets a year, as compared with the usual 13 packs. Since for the 30 μg pills used this will obviously add to the annual ingested dose, it cannot be expected to reduce the risks of major or minor side effects – though the prospective user may be advised that there is also no evidence that it will significantly increase them.

However, there are promising studies of much lower doses (20 μg EE, such as Loestrin 20) in progress, along with absolutely continuous (365/365) pill-taking. So far, these are demonstrating acceptable bleeding patterns for most users (including no bleeding at all in a majority of subjects) – yet this regimen means that *less* artificial estrogen is taken per year than with Microgynon 30 taken the ordinary way. Therefore *on a named patient basis* (p. 150), selected patients who wish to do so may try taking Loestrin 20 continuously.

Clinical implications

For many years, in the short term, the gap between packets of monophasic brands has often been omitted at the woman's choice, to avoid a 'period' on special occasions. Users of phasic pills who wish to postpone withdrawal bleeds must use the final phase of a spare packet, or pills from an equivalent formulation, e.g. Norimin in the case of TriNovum (Janssen–Cilag) or Microgynon 30 immediately after the last tablet of Logynon (Schering Health Care).

In the longer term, in addition to the woman's choice, there exist some special indications for using a tricycle regimen:

Indications for a tricycling regimen (e.g. that shown in Figure 9) using a monophasic pill (in the last three instances (ONLY), the PFI should be shortened to 4 days)

- Woman's choice
- Headaches, including migraine without aura – and other bothersome symptoms – if they occur regularly in the withdrawal week
- Unacceptably heavy or painful withdrawal bleeds
- Paradoxically, to help women who are concerned about absent withdrawal bleeds (less frequent pregnancy tests for reassurance!)
- Premenstrual syndrome – tricycling helps if COCs are used for this
- Endometriosis, where after primary therapy a progestogen-dominant monophasic pill may be tricycled (or, even better, given 365/365) for maintenance treatment
- Epilepsy, which benefits from relatively more sustained levels of the administered hormones, and tricycling with a shortened PFI may also be indicated by the (enzyme-inducing) therapy given
- Long-term enzyme-inducer therapy (discussed below)
- Wherever there is suspicion of decreased efficacy (see above).

Breakthrough bleeding (BTB) may become an unacceptable problem during tricycling, implying that the COC for that woman is unable to maintain endometrial stability for so long. One solution, provided a minimum of seven tablets have been taken

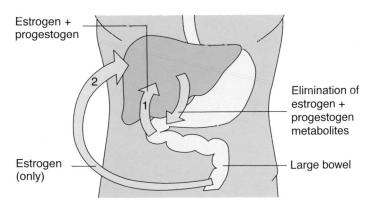

Figure 10
The enterohepatic recirculation of estrogen: (1) 'first-pass' – absorption of hormones in the liver; (2) 'second-pass' – reabsorption of active estrogen (not progestogen).

since the last PFI (and it will usually be far more) is to advise a definite 4- to 7-day break. This sometimes 'clears the decks' so that the BTB stops once the next new course of active tablets commences. Some women tolerate *bicycling* best, i.e. 42 days of continuous pill-taking, followed (depending on the indication) by a 4- to 7-day PFI.

Drug interactions

Interacting drugs reduce the efficacy of COCs mainly by induction of liver enzymes, which leads to increased elimination of both estrogen and progestogen (Figure 10). Additionally, in a very small (but unknown) minority of women, disturbance by certain antibiotics of the gut flora that normally split estrogen metabolites that arrive in the bowel can reduce the reabsorption of some reactivated estrogen. According to WHOMEC, this effect is probably negligible clinically (but see below). It is definitely not a factor in the maintenance of progestogen levels, and so is irrelevant to the POP. The most clinically important drugs with which interaction occurs are given below.

Enzyme-inducer drugs (important examples) that interact with COCs
- Rifampicin, rifabutin
- Griseofulvin (antifungal)
- Barbiturates
- Phenytoin
- Carbamazepine
- Oxcarbazepine
- Primidone
- Topiramate (if daily dose >200 mg)
- Modafinil
- Some antiretrovirals (e.g. ritonavir, nevirapine) – full details are obtainable from www.hiv-druginteractions.org
- St John's Wort – potency of shop-bought product varies enormously; CSM advises *non-use* with COC or POP

Non-liver enzyme-inducing antibiotics that might possibly interact with COCs

These are not listed, since, on pragmatic and in part on medicolegal grounds, the Faculty of FP now recommends that the short-term advice below be given for *all* antimicrobial drugs. In some cases, this is overly cautious: co-trimoxazole, erythromycin and clarithromycin for example actually tend to raise blood levels of EE, although there is no evidence of consequential thrombotic risk (grapefruit juice is similar!).

Other relevant drugs

Note that none of the proton-pump inhibitors – including *lansoprazole* – are now regarded as having any clinically important enzyme-induction effect. Moreover *ethosuximide*, *valproate and clonazepam* and most newer anti-epileptic drugs (including *vigabatrin* and *lamotrigine*) do not pose this COC-efficacy-reducing problem.

- *Lamotrigine* levels can be *lowered* by COCs, so starting a COC in a patient already taking this drug may result in poorer control of the epilepsy: awareness and a small increment in the dose of lamotrigine is all that is required. Moreover, on aware of the same *possibility* with all progestogen-only methods (but no good data).
    - There is no problem in giving lamotrigine to patients already taking a COC, because the dose of anti-epileptic drug is as usual titrated to the patient's needs.
    - However the lamotrigine dose may need to be lowered when the COC is discontinued.
- *Ciclosporin* levels can be *raised* by COC hormones: the risk of toxic effects means blood levels should be measured.
- *Potassium-sparing diuretics* there is a risk of *hyperkalaemia* with drospirenone, the progestogen in *Yasmin*, so these diuretics should not be used (WHO 4) with that COC.

Clinical Implications

Short-term use of *any* interacting drug (enzyme-inducer or antibiotic)

Recommended regimen

- Additional contraceptive precautions are advised during the treatment, and should then be continued for a further 7 days.
- If at the end of treatment there are fewer than seven tablets left in the pack (i.e. the third week), the next PFI should be eliminated (skip any placebo pills).
- *Rifampicin* is such a powerful enzyme inducer that even if it is given only for 2 days (e.g. to eliminate carriage of meningococci), increased COC elimination by the liver must be assumed for 4 weeks thereafter, i.e. as though it had been given long term (see below). The extra contraception (e.g. condoms) should therefore be continued to cover all that time, together *also* with the elimination of any expected PFIs.

Longer-term use of antimicrobials

The large-bowel flora responsible for recycling estrogens are reconstituted with resistant organisms within about 2 weeks. In practice, therefore, if COCs are commenced in a woman who has been taking a tetracycline long-term, there is no need to advise extra contraceptive precautions. There is a potential problem (now believed to involve very few women – but clinically we never know which) in the reverse situation, i.e. when the tetracycline is first introduced to treat a long-term COC user. Even then:

- Extra precautions need only be sustained for a maximum of 21 days, which includes the usual 7 days for ovarian suppression, along with:
- Elimination of the next PFI if the 2 weeks of antimicrobial use involved any of the last seven pills of a pack.

Long-term use of enzyme-inducers

This applies chiefly to epileptic women and women being treated for tuberculosis. This situation is WHO 3, meaning that an alternative method of contraception is preferable – especially for those on rifampicin or rifabutin, whose adverse effects on efficacy of the COC are such that long-term users are strongly advised against it. Relevant options that should *always first be discussed* are the injectable DMPA (with *no special advice* now needed to shorten the injection interval), an IUD or LNG-IUS.

If the combined Pill is nevertheless chosen:

Recommended regimen
- Prescribe an increased dose, usually 50–60 µg estrogen by taking two tablets daily, and also:
- Advise one of the tricycle regimens described above (this is particularly appropriate for epileptic women, since the frequency of attacks is often reduced by the maintenance of steady hormone levels), and also:
- The PFI should be shortened at the end of each tricycle: such that the next packet is started after 4 days, even if the withdrawal bleed has not stopped.

Only one 50 µg pill remains on the UK market (Table 2) and metabolic conversion of the prodrug mestranol to EE is only about 75% efficient. Therefore Norinyl-1 is almost identical to Norimin. So the Faculty of FP recommends constructing a 50 or

60 µg regimen from two sub 50 µg products, e.g. two tablets daily of Microgynon 30, or a Femodene (Schering Health Care) plus a Femodette tablet (see Table 2). As this practice is unlicensed, this is named-patient use and the guidance on p. 150 should be followed. The woman can be reassured that she is metaphorically 'climbing a down escalator' so as to stay in the right place – her increased liver metabolism means that her body should still in reality be receiving a normal low-dose regimen.

Breakthrough bleeding and interacting drugs

BTB may occur – indeed, it could have been the first clue to a drug interaction. If the long-term user of an enzyme-inducer develops persistent BTB, the first step is to exclude another cause (see the checklist box on p. 57). Then recommend a 4- to 7-day break in the continuous tablet-taking. If the problem persists after recommencing tablets, a change of method will nearly always be preferable. The alternative of trying an even higher dose, combining pills to a total estrogen content of say 80–90 µg in an attempt to increase the blood levels of both hormones to above the threshold for bleeding, is not now recommended, given some uncertainty about VTE risk (even with the enzyme induction occurring).

Discontinuation of enzyme-inducers after long-term use

It has been shown that 4 or more weeks may elapse before excretory function in the liver reverts to normal. Hence, if any of these drugs has been used for 1–2 months (or at all in the case of rifampicin/rifabutin), there should be a delay of about 4 weeks before returning to a standard low-dose regimen. This period should be increased to 8 weeks after more prolonged use of enzyme-inducers. In all cases, there should be no PFI gap between the higher-dose and low-dose packets.

Counselling and ongoing supervision

Starting the COC

After taking a full personal and family history, with full consideration of possible contraindications on the WHO 1–4 scale, as described above, each woman deserves individual teaching, backed (as well as by the manufacturer's patient information leaflet, PIL) by the FPA's user-friendly leaflet *Your Guide to the*

Table 7
Starting routines for COCs

Conditions before start	Start when?	Extra precautions for 7 days
1. Menstruating	On Day 1 or 2 of period	No[a]
	On Day 3 or later	Yes
	Any time in cycle (Quick Start)	Yes[b]
2. Postpartum (a) No lactation	Day 21[c] (low risk of thrombosis: first ovulation reported after Day 28)	No
(b) Lactation	Not normally recommended (POP or injectable preferred)	
3. After induced abortion/miscarriage	Same day or Day 2 (Day 21 if beyond 24 weeks' gestation)	No
4. After trophoblastic tumour	1 month after no hCG detected	As **1.**
5. After higher dose COC	Instant switch or use condoms after PFI for 7 days[d]	No
6. After lower or same-dose COC	After usual 7-day break	No
7. After POP	First day of period	No
8. During POP-induced secondary amenorrhoea	Any day (end of packet)	No
9. Other secondary amenorrhoea including after DMPA (pregnancy excluded)[e]	Any day	Yes
10. First period after postcoital contraception	By Day 2 when woman sure her flow is normal *or* Quick Start[b], i.e. immediately (see p. 131)	No Yes

Note that there are some differences here from UKMEC.

[a]ED pill users also start with the first *active* pill on day 1. By applying the right sticky strip (out of seven supplied) for that weekday, all future pills are then labelled with the correct days. A useful alternative is 'Sunday start', in which the woman takes the first active pill on the 1st Sunday after her period starts, with condom use sustained until 7 active pills have been taken (this ensures that from then onwards there are no bleeds at weekends).

[b]'Quick Start' means starting any day provided the prescriber is satisfied there has been no earlier conception risk that cycle (see also p. 145).

[c]Puerperal risk lasts longer after *severe* pregnancy-related hypertension, or the related HELLP syndrome (haemolysis, elevated liver enzymes, low platelets), so delay COC use until the return of normal BP and biochemistry. This history in the past is WHO 1.

[d]If usual 7-day break, rebound ovulation may occur at the time of transfer.

[e]Meaning prescriber is confident that no blastocyst or sperm is already in the upper genital tract, if necessary through a negative sensitive pregnancy test after at least 14 days of safe contraception or abstinence from intercourse. See pp. 145–6.

Combined Pill. After dealing with the woman's concerns and any questions she may have about risks and benefits – particularly about cancer and circulatory disease – and about 'minor' side effects, the recommended starting routines should be followed as in Table 7. Note the important footnotes.

She should be advised about maintaining sexual health: if now or at some time in the future she is not in a mutually monogamous relationship, she should be warned to use condoms (ideally supplied on the spot), in addition to the COC or other 'medical' method. The main take-home messages to be conveyed to a new user are summarized below.

Take-home messages for a new Pill-taker

- *Your FPA leaflet:* this is not to be read and thrown away, it is something to keep safely in a drawer somewhere, for ongoing reference.
- *The Pill only works if you take it correctly:* if you do, each new pack will always start on the same day of the week.
- *Even if bleeding, like a 'period', occurs (BTB), carry on Pill-taking:* ring for advice if necessary. Nausea is another common early symptom. Both usually settle as your body gets used to the Pill.
- ***Never be a late restarter of your Pill!*** Even if your 'period' (withdrawal bleed) has not stopped yet, never start your next packet late. This is because the PFI is obviously a time when your contraceptive is not being supplied to your ovaries, so they might anyway be beginning to escape from its actions.
- *Lovemaking during the 7 days after any packet is only safe if you do actually go on to the next pack.* Otherwise (e.g. if you decide to stop the method) you must start using condoms after the last Pill in the pack.
- For what to do if any Pill(s) *are* more than 24 hours late, see p. 46.
- Other things that may stop the Pill from working include *vomiting* and *some drugs* (always mention that you are on the Pill).
- See a doctor *at once* if any of the things on p. 61 occur, especially new headaches with strange *changes in your eyesight happening beforehand.*
- *As a one-off, you can shorten one PFI* to make sure all your future withdrawal bleeds avoid weekends.
- *You can avoid bleeding on holidays etc.* by running packs together. (Discuss this with whoever provides your Pills, if you want to continue missing out 'periods' long term.)
- Good though it is as a contraceptive, *the Pill does not give enough protection against Chlamydia and other STIs*. Whenever in doubt, especially with a new partner, use a condom *as well.*
- Finally, *always feel free to telephone or come back at any time* (maybe to the practice nurse) for any reasons of your own, including any symptoms you would like dealt with.

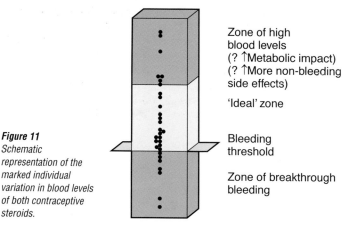

Zone of high
blood levels
(? ↑Metabolic impact)
(? ↑More non-bleeding
side effects)

'Ideal' zone

Bleeding
threshold

Zone of breakthrough
bleeding

Figure 11
*Schematic
representation of the
marked individual
variation in blood levels
of both contraceptive
steroids.*

Second choice of Pill brand

How this relates to the symptom of breakthrough bleeding

Some women react unpredictably, and it is a false expectation that any single Pill will suit all women. Individual variations in motivation and tolerance of minor side-effects are well recognized. But, due to differences in absorption and metabolism, there is also marked variability (threefold, in the area under the curve) in *blood levels of the exogenous hormones* (Figure 11). This is relevant to the management of irregular bleeding.

Bleeding side effects

Given the 'model' shown in Figure 11 by the variability of blood levels and BTB risk, prescribers should try to identify the lowest dose for each woman that does not cause BTB. This should minimize adverse side effects, both serious and minor, and also reduce measurable metabolic changes. Since COCs all have a powerful contraceptive effect, this approach does not appear to impair effectiveness (far more important is not lengthening the PFI; see above). Even if BTB occurs, provided there is ongoing good compliance with Pill-taking, extra contraception (e.g. with condoms) does not need to be advised.

- The objective is that each woman should receive the least long-term metabolic impact that her uterus will allow, i.e.

the lowest dose of contraceptive steroids that is just – but only just – above her bleeding threshold.
- If BTB does occur and is unacceptable or persists beyond two cycles, a different or higher dose brand should be tried, though only **after** the checks in the checklist below. Phasic COCs are generally second-choice formulations, but they are certainly worth trying here for BTB (and also for the symptom of absence of withdrawal bleeding).

It is vital to exclude other causes of BTB before blaming the COC!

Checklist for abnormal bleeding in a Pill-user[a]
- **DISEASE:** Consider examining the cervix (it is not unknown for bleeding from an invasive cancer to be wrongly attributed, and any bloodstained discharge should always trigger the thought '*Chlamydia?*').
- **DISORDERS of PREGNANCY** that cause bleeding (e.g. retained products if the COC was started after a recent termination of pregnancy).
- **DEFAULT:** BTB may be triggered 2 or 3 days after missed Pills and may be persistent thereafter.
- **DRUGS**, primarily enzyme-inducers (see text). Cigarettes are also drugs in this context: BTB is statistically more common among smokers.
- **Diarrhoea** and/or **VOMITING:** Diarrhoea alone has to be exceptionally severe to impair absorption significantly.
- **DISTURBANCES of ABSORPTION:** for example after massive gut resection.
- **DURATION of USE too short:** i.e. assessment is too early (minimal BTB that is tolerable for longer may then cease after 3 months use of any new formulation). The opposite possibility may apply during tricycling (see pp. 47), namely that the duration of continuous use has been too long for that woman's endometrium to be sustained, in which case a *bleeding-triggered* 4- to 7-day break may be taken; or bicycling of two packets in a row may be substituted.
- **DOSE:** after the above have been excluded, it is possible to try a phasic Pill if the woman is receiving monophasic treatment; increase the progestogen component (or of the estrogen, if a 20 μg COC is in use); try a different progestogen.

[a]Modified from Sapire E. *Contraception and Sexuality in Health and Disease*. New York: McGraw-Hill, 1990.

Second choice of Pill if there are non-bleeding side effects

- When symptoms occur, it is generally bad practice to give further prescriptions to control them without changing the COC – such as diuretics for weight gain or antidepressants for mood symptoms.

Which second choice of pill? Relative oestrogen excess	
Symptoms • Nausea • Dizziness • Cyclical weight gain (fluid), 'bloating' – Yasmin is also worth a try here despite its estrogenicity, given the anti-mineralo-corticoid activity of drospirenone • Vaginal discharge (no infection) • Some cases of breast enlargement/pain • Some cases of lost libido without depression, especially if taking an anti-androgen (Yasmin or Dianette)	**Conditions** • Benign breast disease • Fibroids • Endometriosis
Treat with progestogen-dominant COC, such as Microgynon 30 (Schering Health Care). Loestrin 20 is an oestrogen-deficient option	

Which second choice of pill? Relative progestogen excess	
Symptoms • Dryness of vagina • Some cases of sustained weight gain – although there is actuallt no ghood evidence that modern COCs cause the weight gain for which they are often blamed • Depression/lassitude • Depressed mood ± associated loss of libido • Breast tenderness	**Conditions** • Acne/seborrhoea • Hirsutism
Treat with oestrogen-dominant COC, such as Marvelon (Organon Laboratories) or in moderately severe cases of acne or hirsutism, Yasmin or Dianette (see text). Note that caution is necessary, in that oestrogen dominance may correlate with a slightly higher risk of VTE, especially in, for example obesity (Table 5)].	

- There are two main preferred, if empirical, courses of action:
  - to decrease the dose of either hormone, if possible (in the limit, estrogen can be eliminated by a trial of a POP); or
  - to change to a different progestogen.
- Additionally, although the evidence is mainly anecdotal, there is a little guidance available for side effects and conditions associated with a relative excess of either steroid.

More about Yasmin

Acne, seborrhoea and sometimes hirsutism may be benefited by any of the estrogen-dominant COCs. Yasmin is a monophasic COC containing 3 mg drospironone (DSP) and 30 μg EE. DSP differs from other progestogens in COCs because:

- It acts as an anti-androgen, so the combination is an alternative to Dianette for the treatment of moderately severe acne and PCOS.
- It has diuretic properties due to anti-mineralocorticoid activity.

Yasmin is a useful choice for appropriate women, for example:
- A clear indication for estrogen/anti-androgen therapy, such as moderately severe acne (Marvelon works well for milder cases), including cases associated with PCOS.
- As a useful second choice for empirical control of minor side effects: particularly those associated with fluid retention such as bloatedness and cyclical breast enlargement. It seems to be of value for women with the premenstrual syndrome, whether in their normal cycle or also occurring on another COC – in which case continuous use or tricycling is preferable.
- Last, and definitely least, what about weight? In one study, there was a maintained slight (about 1%) reduction of body mass, but probably due only to less total body water compared with controls. Also, if the BMI is already above 30, there is a safety issue for any COC – although if it is being given for therapy, the risk–benefit analysis may be different (see p. 32).
- *Anxiety* about weight, or a history of fluid retention-linked weight gain with previously used COCs, would justify a trial of Yasmin.

Where does Dianette feature now?

This is another anti-androgen plus estrogen combination – cyproterone acetate (CPA) 2 mg with EE 35 μg – licensed for the treatment of moderately severe acne and mild hirsutism in women. These are its indications, but practically everything about the COC in this book applies also to Dianette: it is a reliable anovulant, usually giving good cycle control, and has similar rules for missed tablets, interactions, absolute and relative contraindications, and requirements for monitoring.

There has been no good head-to-head randomized controlled trial of Yasmin versus Dianette reported, but indirect evidence suggests that Yasmin would have at least as good effectiveness for the conditions for which Dianette is indicated, and so might usefully be used from the outset. Both are estrogen-dominant products requiring careful assessment of VTE risk factors. An increased VTE risk compared with LNG pills has in fact been shown, as might be expected, for Dianette, but *not* so far for Yasmin (EURAS study).

Duration of treatment with Dianette needs to be individualized. In the SPC (data sheet), it is recommended that 'treatment is withdrawn when the acne or hirsutism is completely resolved', but 'repeat courses may be given if the condition recurs'. There are some concerns related to hepatic effects (not confirmed, and very small if real).

Clinical implications

Unless there are particularly strong *therapeutic* indications for the use of Dianette rather than Yasmin (whose SPC mentions no particular duration limits), it is usual.

- To encourage patients to switch when their condition is controlled, perhaps after about 1 year, commonly to Marvelon. The latter can be promoted to the woman as likely to be quite sufficient as *maintenance* treatment for what should now be well-controlled acne.
- If there is a relapse, try Yasmin, or:
- Exceptionally, it may be appropriate to return to use of Dianette for much longer.

Stopping COCs

The first menstruation after stopping COCs (for any reason) is often delayed by up to about 6–8 weeks. Secondary amenorrhoea for 6 months should always be investigated, whether or not it occurs after stopping COCs – the link will be coincidental and not causal. Whatever the diagnosis, any associated estrogen deficiency should always be treated.

Listed below are the (only) reasons for discontinuing COCs immediately or soon, and should be understood by all well-counselled women from their first visit (similar lists are in most PILs, and in the FPA's recommended leaflet *Your Guide to the Combined Pill*). The worst implications of these symptoms are Pill-related thrombotic or embolic catastrophes in the making. Often there is another explanation, and the COC may be recommenced later. Pending diagnosis, the COC, because of its contained EE, should be stopped, but any progestogen-only method (e.g. Cerazette) could be started immediately.

Symptoms for which COCs should be stopped immediately, pending investigation and treatment
- Unusual or severe and very prolonged headache
- Diagnosis of aura (see above), usually involving loss of part or whole of the field of vision on one side; or (unrelated to migraine) loss of sight in one eye
- Disturbance of speech (nominal dysphasia in migraine with aura)
- Numbness, severe paraesthesia or weakness on one side of the body, e.g. one arm, side of the tongue; indeed, any symptom suggesting cerebral ischaemia or TIA
- A severe unexplained fainting attack or severe acute vertigo or ataxia
- Focal epilepsy
- Painful swelling in the calf
- Pain in the chest, especially pleuritic pain
- Breathlessness or cough with bloodstained sputum
- Severe abdominal pain
- Immobilization, for example:
  - after most lower limb fractures or
  - *major* surgery or
  - leg surgery.

In all the above circumstances, stop COC and consider anti-thrombotic treatment. If an elective procedure is planned and the Pill stopped more than 2 weeks ahead (4 weeks is preferable), anticoagulation is not usually necessary. Contraception can be maintained nowadays by switching to and then later from Cerazette, which is believed to have negligible pro-thrombotic effects.

Pill follow-up: What is important?

Aside from the management of established risk factors or diseases already present, or that may suddenly or more gradually appear, and of new minor side-effects (both dealt with above), follow-up primarily entails two items of monitoring:

- blood pressure (BP)
- headaches, especially migraine.

Blood pressure

Monitoring of BP is vital. It should be recorded before COCs are started and checked after 3 months (1 month in a high-risk case) and subsequently at intervals of 6 months. After about 15 months (UKMEC proposes this as soon as after the 3 month visit), if there is no rise between successive measurements, the interval can reasonably be increased to annually in women without risk factors. COCs should always be stopped altogether if BP exceeds 160/95 mmHg on repeated measurements (p. 00). A more moderate increase still suggests the possibility of an increased risk of arterial disease, especially in the presence of any other arterial risk factors (see Table 6). But, in the opinion of WHOMEC and UKMEC, it should now be the norm for normotensive women to receive a year's supply of the COC at a time (so long as it is made abundantly clear that they may return sooner for advice, as they may wish – an 'open-house' policy).

Headaches

Not to ask about a COC-taker's headaches at the regular pill follow-up visit would be a serious omission: see above for the crucial importance of identifying migraine with aura.

Screening

Note what is **not** included above in the follow-up requirements: neither breast and bimanual pelvic examinations nor monitoring blood tests have any relevance to Pill follow-up. *Routine* biman-ual pelvic examinations in asymptomatic COC-takers are partic-ularly uncalled for, because the disorders causing detectable pelvic masses or tenderness are, as listed on p. 13, all actually *less frequent* in COC-takers than in others.

Even taking cervical smears is for screening and not a COC-associated exercise. After the age of 25, cervical screening should simply be performed regularly, as guidelines recommend for all sexually active women.

Congenital abnormalities and fertility issues

Any possible effect of COCs on congenital abnormalities is hard to establish because it is so difficult to prove a negative; moreover, 2% of all full-term fetuses have a significant malfor-mation.

- Even with exposure during organogenesis, meta-analyses of the major studies fail to show an increased risk. If present it must be very small.
- Used *prior to* the conception cycle, the conclusions of a WHO scientific group have not since been challenged – namely, that there is no good evidence for any adverse effects on the fetus of COCs. It can do no harm if a woman stops COCs and switches to barriers for 2 or more months before conception, but there is no objective evidence that it is worth the effort. Certainly, any woman who finds herself pregnant immediately after stopping COCs should be strongly reassured.

What about 'taking breaks' to optimize fertility?

Concerns about its reversibility have dogged the COC since its first marketing. Fertile ovulation can be minimally delayed on cessation, for a matter of days or up to 4 weeks – a much shorter time than following injectable use (see below). Yet, just as for the latter method, there is no evidence that COCs can cause permanent loss of fertility. Indeed, a large study by Farrow et al (*Hum Reprod* 2002; **17**: 2754–61) showed that use of the COC for more than 5 years before the 8497 *planned* conceptions was associated with a *decreased* risk of delay in conceiving, even for nulliparous women!

If a woman still feels more comfortable to take a routine break from the COC, we should always help her to find a satisfactory contraceptive alternative. However, there is no known benefit:

- to fertility or
- to health

from taking short elective breaks of 6 months or so every few years, as was once recommended. It helps some women to be reminded that regular PFIs give the body plenty of breaks from the COC anyway, totalling 130 every 10 years!

In one study, a quarter of young women who took breaks as above had unwanted conceptions. Relevantly, another finding of the Farrow et al study quoted above was that one-third of the whole population admitted their pregnancy was not truly planned – and this was a large population surveyed in *antenatal clinics*, and thus could not include those others who had pregnancies terminated.

Summary
- The first visit for prescription of COCs is by far the most important, and should never be rushed.
- The LARCs, long-term and 'forgettable' contraceptive options should always be included in the discussion, despite the woman's presenting request for what she happens to know about (most probably the Pill).
- If the Pill remains her choice, along with discussing the risks and benefits, and fully assessing her medical and family history – all at her level of understanding – there is much ground to cover (see the Take-Home Messages list above). Often it is useful to share this between the doctor and practice or clinic nurse.
- Thereafter, there are really only three key components to COC monitoring during follow-up:
  - BP
  - headaches
  - identification and management of any new risk factors/diseases/side effects.

No matter how carefully those with contraindications are excluded, a few women will experience adverse effects. Repeated presentation with multiple side effects sometimes suggests the offer of a different method rather than a different pill, or – if anxiety about possible adverse effects seems excessive – that there is a hidden psychosexual problem.

TRANSDERMAL COMBINED HORMONAL CONTRACEPTION

Evra

Evra (Janssen-Cilag) is an innovative transdermal patch delivering EE with norelgestromin, the active metabolite of NGM. In some ways, it can be seen as 'transdermal Cilest'. The daily skin dose of 150 µg norelgestromin and 20 µg EE produces blood levels in the reference range of those after a tablet of Cilest, but without either the latter's diurnal fluctuations or the oral peak dose given to the liver. Pending more specific research information, all the absolute and relative contraindications and indeed most of the above practical management advice about the COC apply, with obvious minor adjustments, to this new product. It appears to be relatively quite estrogen-dominant, with a bleeding and non-bleeding side-effect profile very like Cilest itself – in addition, about 2% of women in the trials had local skin reactions that led to discontinuation.

The patch has generally good adhesion even in hot climates and when bathing or showering: the incidence of detachment of patches was 1.8% (complete) and 2.9% (partial). In the pooled analysis of the randomized controlled trials, the failure rate for consistent users of Evra was similar to that of the oral pills – less than 1 per 100 woman-years. Interestingly, in the clinical trials, one-third of the few failures occurred in the 3% of the population who weighed above 90 kg. This apparently reduced effectiveness contraindicates (WHO 4) Evra for such women, who are at minimum WHO 3 for VTE risk at that level of BMI anyway and far from ideal users of an estrogen-dominant product.

Maintenance of efficacy of Evra
- Avoid use at all if body weight >90 kg.
- Warn the user that the contraceptive is in the glue of the patch, so a dry patch that has fallen off should not be re-used!
- Each patch is worn for 7 days, for 3 consecutive weeks followed by a patch-free week. This regimen was shown to aid compliance, particularly in young women. Under age 20, perfect use was reported by COC users in 68% of cycles, but in 88% of cycles by patch-users.

Clinically, the patch is therefore a useful alternative to offer to those who find it difficult to remember a daily pill, especially as, if the patch-user does forget, there is a 2-day margin for error for late patch change. Setting up a weekly text-message reminder 'Today is your patch-change day' can also be very helpful!

- As with the COC, it is essential never to lengthen the contraception-free (patch-free) interval.
- If this interval *exceeds* 8 days for any reason (either through late application or through the first new patch detaching and this being identified late), advise extra precautions for the duration of the first freshly applied patch (i.e. for 7 days). EC should be considered if there has been sexual exposure during the preceding patch-free time, particularly if that exceeded 9 days.
- Absorption problems through vomiting/diarrhoea, and tetracycline by mouth, have no effect on this method's efficacy, but:
- During any short-term enzyme-inducer therapy, and for 28 days after this ends, additional contraception (e.g. with condoms) is advised, plus elimination of any patch-free intervals during this time.

TRANSVAGINAL COMBINED HORMONAL CONTRACEPTION

Already available in several European countries and the USA, NuvaRing (Organon) is expected in the UK during 2008. It is a combined vaginal ring that releases etonogestrel (3-ketodesogestrel) 120 μg and EE 15 μg per day, thus equating to some degree with 'vaginal Mercilon'. It is normally retained (though there is an unrestricted option to remove it for up to 3 hours during sexual activity) for 3 weeks and then taken out for a withdrawal bleed during the fourth.

Pending more dedicated information, all the absolute and relative contraindications, and most of the above practical management advice about the COC, apply also to NuvaRing. It appears to be relatively estrogen-dominant, with a side-effect profile very like that of Mercilon itself. In studies, it proved very popular, with excellent cycle control and once again a failure rate comparable to that of the COC.

Maintenance of efficacy of NuvaRing

- Expulsions were a problem for some (usually parous) women, primarily during the emptying of bowels or bladder, and therefore readily recognized.
- As with the COC, it will still be essential never to lengthen the contraception-free (ring-free) interval. If for any reason this exceeds 8 days, advise extra precautions for 7 days. As for Evra, EC should be considered if there has been sexual exposure during any ring-free time, particularly if that exceeded 9 days.
- Absorption problems, vomiting/diarrhoea and broad-spectrum antibiotics apparently have no detectable effect on this method's efficacy.
- During any short-term enzyme-inducer therapy, and for 28 days after this ends, additional contraception (e.g. with condoms) is advised, plus elimination of any ring-free intervals during this time.

Progestogen-only pill

There are five varieties of progestogen-only pill (POP) available (Table 8): four are of the old type that variably inhibit ovulation, while the fifth, Cerazette, is a primarily anovulant product. The latter is very different and therefore is mainly dealt with at the end of this section. Unless otherwise stated the abbreviation POP will refer to the four old-type POPs.

Table 8
Available POPs

Product	Constituents	Course of treatment
Noriday	350 µg norethisterone	28 tablets
Micronor	350 µg norethisterone	28 tablets
Femulen	500 µg etynodiol diacetate	28 tablets
Norgeston	30 µg levonorgestrel	35 tablets
Cerazette	75 µg desogestrel	28 tablets

Mechanism of action and maintenance of effectiveness

The mechanism of action is complex because of variable interactions between the administered progestogen and the endogenous activity of the woman's ovary. Outside of lactation (when their effectiveness is hugely enhanced, see below), fertile ovulation is prevented in 50–60% of cycles. In the remainder, there is reliance mainly on *progestogenic interference with mucus penetrability*. This 'barrier' effect is readily lost, so that each tablet daily must be taken within 3 hours of the same regular time.

If POPs are indeed taken regularly each day within that time span of 27 hours, without breaks and regardless of bleeding patterns, they are in practice as effective (or as ineffective, in 'typical use, see Table 1!) as COCs – especially for those aged 35 and over.

Effectiveness

In the UK, the Oxford/FPA study reported a failure rate of 3.1 per 100 woman-years between the ages 25 and 29, but this improved to 1.0 at 35–39 years of age and was as low as 0.3 for women over 40 years of age. Realistically, most users are probably not as meticulous as those married middle-class women.

With regard to effect of body mass (not BMI), studies are suggestive, but not conclusive, that the failure rate of old-type POPs may be higher with increasing weight, as was well established in early studies of progestogen rings and some implants. Pending more data, a logical policy now is to use Cerazette as first choice for women over 70 kg (irrespective of height), especially if they are young. This is preferable to taking two POPs, though that is still an option off-licence. Because of reduced fertility one POP suffices anyway during established breastfeeding or in older overweight women, above the age of 45.

Missed pills

Interference with contraceptive activity through missed pills, vomiting or drug interaction is believed to start within as little as 3 hours, but is corrected adequately (as far as the mucus is concerned) if renewed Pill-taking is combined with extra precautions for just 48 hours (WHOSPR).

> **Clinically**, after missing a POP for more than 3 hours (or more than 12 hours for Cerazette; see below) the woman should:
>
> - take that day's pill immediately and the next one on time
> - use added precautions for the next 2 days
>
> Additionally, with old-type POPs, if there has already been *intercourse without added protection between the time of first potential loss of the mucus effect through to its restoration by 48 hours, it is appropriate to:*
>
> - advise immediate EC with levonorgestrel (see p. 124), with the next old-type POP being taken on time.

What EC action is necessary during full lactation taking ordinary POPs, or for Cerazette-users (who have 12 hours of 'leeway' anyway?)

Here there is established anovulation (without any of the COC's pill-free intervals, with their contraception-weakening effect). So only the first two bullets above would apply and emergency contraception (EC) would be unnecessary in most cases. Pending more data it could be given on a 'fail-safe' basis for complete omissions of more than one POP during lactation (i.e. beyond 24 hours).

Lactation and the POP

According to the lactational amenorrhoea mathod (LAM – see Figure 19, p. 143), even without the POP, there is only about a 2% conception risk if all three LAM criteria continue to apply.

> **LAM criteria**
> - amenorrhoea, since the lochia ceased
> - full lactation – the baby's nutrition is effectively all from its mother
> - baby not yet 6 months old.

This is why, on any POP during full lactation, postcoital contraception is very rarely indicated for missed POPs. But because breastfeeding varies in its intensity, if a tablet is 3 hours late it is still usual to advise additional precautions during the next two tablet-taking days. See above regarding when, if ever, to give EC.

What dose to the baby?

During lactation, with all POPs (including Cerazette), the dose to the infant is believed to be harmless, but this aspect must always be discussed. The least amount of administered progestogen gets into the breast milk if an LNG POP (Norgeston) is used. The quantity is the equivalent of one POP in 2 years – considerably less than the progesterone of cow's milk origin found in formula feeds.

If EC is required (rather rarely – see above) by a breastfeeding mother, very little LNG reaches the breast milk. She may wish to express and discard her breast milk for 8–12 hours, the dose reaching her baby becoming negligible thereafter.

Weaning

Beware – unwanted conceptions are common when lactating POP-users have not been adequately warned that their margin for error in POP-taking will diminish at weaning. If efficacy is at a premium, they should be given a 'stronger' method, such as a supply of the COC or Cerazette (unless that was already the POP being used in lactation), to start when their infant first takes solid food, or no later than the first bleed.

Drug interactions (Re lamotrigine, see p. 51)

- **Broad-spectrum antibiotics.** These do not interfere with the effectiveness of POPs or indeed any progestogen-only method.
- **Enzyme-inducers.** Another highly effective contraceptive method is advised during use of liver enzyme-inducers such as rifampicin or carbamazepine and, as necessary, for 4 weeks or more even after stopping (see the section on COCs). Long-term treatment with enzyme-inducers is WHO 3, but if a suitable alternative contraceptive is not identified and the couple do not wish to use condoms indefinitely, increasing the dose is an option (my view, not UKMEC) – usually to two POPs or two Cerazettes, daily, the choice depending on all relevant factors including lactation and the woman's body weight, age and likely fertility. This is unlicensed use (p. 150).
- **Bosentan.** This endothelin antagonist is a particular enzyme-inducer drug that would never be relevant for the COC, since it is used to treat pulmonary hypertension (which is WHO 4 for the COC). However, Cerazette (see below) could be a very

appropriate contraceptive for a young woman with this serious condition, in which pregnancy can be lethal – again with two tablets being taken daily to compensate for the enzyme induction. See also p. 150, regarding this whole section, as this double-dosing use is unlicensed.

Risks and disadvantages

Healthwise, being EE-free, these are exceptionally safe products. There are negligible changes to most metabolic variables. There is no proven causative link:

- with any tumour (there was a non-significant increase in breast cancer risk in the 1996 Collaborative Group Study (p. 14), which does not currently influence prescribing)
- nor with venous or (less certainly) arterial disease.

Side effects

The main side effect of POPs and Cerazette is irregular bleeding, about which all prospective users should be clearly warned. The irregularity can include *oligo-amenorrhoea*. This occurs more commonly with Cerazette than with other POPs. But, reassuringly, it appears that with all POPs, Cerazette and Implanon, follicle-stimulating hormone (FSH) is not completely suppressed even during the amenorrhoea, which is mainly caused by luteinising hormone (LH) suppression. There is therefore enough follicular activity at the ovary to maintain adequate mid-follicular phase estrogen levels. Pending more data, this means that there is *not* the concern about bone density reduction that exists for DMPA (see below).

For management of side effects during follow-up, see below.

Advantages and indications

The indications (WHO 1 or sometimes WHO 2) for POP or Cerazette use (see also below) are as follows:

Indications for POP or Cerazette use
- Lactation, where the combination even with ordinary POPs is extra-effective – indeed as good as the COC would be in non-breastfeeders

- Side effects with, or recognized contraindications to, the combined pill, in particular where estrogen-related. As EE-free products do not appear to significantly affect blood-clotting mechanisms, POPs may be used by women with a definite past history of VTE and a whole range of disorders predisposing to arterial or venous disease. Good counselling and record-keeping are essential
- Major or leg surgery or over the time of injection treatments for varicose veins – when COCs are contraindicated on VTE grounds
- Sickle cell disease, severe structural heart disease, pulmonary hypertension (Cerazette)
- Smokers above 35 years of age
- Hypertension, whether COC-related or not, controlled on treatment
- Migraine, including varieties with aura (the woman may well continue to suffer migraines, but the fear of an EE-promoted thrombotic stroke is eliminated). Cerazette is preferred, to obtain optimum stability of endogenous hormones whose fluctuation may cause attacks
- Diabetes mellitus (DM) – but caution WHO 3 or 4 if there is significant DM with tissue damage (see the box below)
- Obesity – but then usually prescribing Cerazette (see text)
- At the woman's choice.

Old-type POPs are still good during lactation and for the older woman, given diminished fertility: but for the young highly fertile woman, Cerazette is now the POP of choice.

Problems and contraindications

Absolute contraindications (WHO 4) for POP and Cerazette use
(These are far fewer than for the COC)

- Any serious adverse effect of COCs not certainly related solely to the estrogen (e.g. liver adenoma or cancer, although WHOMEC says WHO 3)
- Recent breast cancer not yet clearly in remission (see below)
- Acute porphyria, if there is a history of actual attack triggered by hormones (progestogens as well as estrogens are believed capable of precipitating these); otherwise WHO 3 (see below)
- Undiagnosed genital tract bleeding
- Actual or possible pregnancy
- Hypersensitivity to any component.

There are also some strong relative contraindications:

Strong relative contraindications (WHO 3) for POP and Cerazette use

- Past *severe* arterial diseases, or current exceptionally high risk
- Sex-steroid-dependent cancer, including breast cancer, when in complete remission (WHOMEC states WHO 4 until 5 years, then WHO 3). In all cases, agreement of the relevant hospital consultant should be obtained and the woman's autonomy respected: record that she understands it is unknown whether progestogen might alter the recurrence risk (either way)
- Recent trophoblastic disease until hCG is undetectable in blood as well as urine (UKMEC; see the section on COCs), but WHO 1 according to WHOMEC – even with high hCG levels
- Enzyme-inducers: although two POPs can be taken, off licence (see above), another method such as an injectable, IUD or LNG-IUS would be preferable
- Acute porphyria, latent, or with no hormone-triggered previous attack (along with caution, forewarning/monitoring); POP is fully usable (WHO 2) in all the non-acute porphyrias
- Past symptomatic (painful) functional ovarian cysts. But persistent cysts/follicles that are commonly detected on routine ultrasonography can be disregarded if they caused no symptoms
- Previous treatment for ectopic pregnancy in a nulliparous woman; however, this is an *indication* for Cerazette! The overall risk of ectopic pregnancy is actually reduced among POP users, which is why the condition is classified by UKMEC as WHO 1. But since the risk can be reduced still further by methods that regularly block fertilization, it would usually be preferable to offer the COC, DMPA, Cerazette or Implanon – to better preserve the precious remaining fallopian tube.

There remain some relative contraindications, where the POP method is generally WHO 2 and so may actually be seen as *indications* when alternatives are rejected:

Weak relative contraindications (WHO 2) for POP and Cerazette use

- Unwillingness to cope with irregularity or absence of periods
- Past VTE or severe risk factors for VTE
- Risk factors for arterial disease – more than one risk factor can be present, in contrast to COCs
- Current liver disorder – even if there is persistent biochemical change

- Most other chronic severe systemic diseases (but WHO 3 if the condition causes significant malabsorption of sex steroids)
- Strong family history of breast cancer – UKMEC says WHO 1 for this – even for COCs in fact! Yet intuitively it seems better in such women to avoid estrogen (and also to give a lower progestogen dose through use of a POP).

Table 9
Starting routines for POPs

Condition before start	Start when?	Extra precautions?
Menstruation	Day 1 of period	No
	Days 2–5	No
	Any time in cycle ('Quick start')	2 days[a]
Postpartum:		
No lactation	Usually Day 21 (can be earlier)	No
Lactation	Day 21 – maybe later if 100% lactation (UKMEC recommends delay till 6 weeks)	No
After induced abortion/ miscarriage	Same day	No
After COCs	Instant switch	No
Amenorrhoea (e.g. postpartum)	Any time[b]	2 days

[a]Can start any day in selected cases **if** the prescriber is satisfied there has been no conception risk up to the starting day.
[b]If prescriber is confident that no blastocyst or sperm is already in upper genital tract (see p. 145).

Counselling and ongoing supervision

The starting routines are summarized in Table 9.

A crucial aspect of counselling is how not to forget – given the 3-hour time window (and only 12 hours with Cerazette). A most useful tip, since almost everyone has a mobile phone, is to routinely advise dedicating one phone alarm to 'POP-taking time'.

Frequent or prolonged menstrual bleeding
This is the main nuisance side effect. With advance warning, it may be tolerated. Improvement appears more likely with

Cerazette, based on the randomized controlled trial comparing it with an LNG POP. By 1 year, around half of ongoing Cerazette users reported amenorrhoea (which with counselling can be accepted as an advantage) or infrequent bleeding (one or two bleeds per 90 days). But the improved bleeding pattern was only evident when users persevered beyond 6 months, and there is no known effective treatment (two tablets daily may be tried) aside from trying a change of POP or a change of method.

A few women experience very prolonged or heavy bleeding, and if – after excluding a non-POP-related, such as gynaecological, cause (see p. 57) – this is not relieved by changing the POP, then another method should be offered.

Amenorrhoea

Except during full lactation, prolonged spells of amenorrhoea occur most often in older women. Once pregnancy has been excluded, the amenorrhoea must be the result of anovulation, and so signifies very high efficacy – as well as convenience for many.

Non-bleeding side-effects

These are rare with POPs, apart from the following complaints:

- *Breast tenderness,* though common, is usually transient; if it recurs, it can sometimes be overcome by changing POPs – especially to Cerazette.
- *Functional cysts* or luteinised unruptured follicles are also not uncommon; however, most are symptomless, and pelvic pain on one or other side is relatively unusual.

Clinically, if functional cysts among POP-users do become symptomatic, they can lead to problems in the differential diagnosis from ectopic pregnancy (pain, menstrual disturbance and a tender adnexal mass being present in both conditions).

Monitoring

The BP of POP-takers is checked initially, but thereafter, if still normal after 1 year, it really does not need to be taken more often than for other women. When raised during COC use, it usually reverts to normal on POPs. Indeed, if it does not, the woman most probably has essential hypertension.

Return of fertility after all POPs, including Cerazette
This is rapid: indeed *clinically,* from the user's point of view, fertility after stopping must be assumed to be immediate.

Menopause
Establishing ovarian failure at the menopause is less important than with the COC, since all the POPs are safe enough products to continue using to the end of the sixth decade. Hence, first switching to any POP from any other hormonal method can be a reassuring way to manage that often difficult transition out of the reproductive years.

On an old-type POP (not the pituitary-suppressing Cerazette), if amenorrhoea develops above the age of 50, a high blood FSH measurement (>30 IU/l) suggests ovarian failure. Two high values 6 weeks apart, especially if there are vasomotor symptoms, would make the likelihood of a later ovulation very low. Should the FSH be found to be low, however, this suggests (despite the amenorrhoea) continuing ovarian function. If the POP is not simply continued to an age when ovarian function must be negligible (p. 148), there would be need for an additional contraceptive – such as condoms, or at this age, 'weaker' methods such as the sponge or spermicide. See p. 139.

Cerazette

Mechanism of action and maintenance of effectiveness
This product contains 75 μg desogestrel and to some extent 'rewrites the text books' about POPs – mainly because it blocks ovulation in 97% of cycles and had a failure rate in the pre-marketing study of only 0.17 per 100 woman-years (in 'perfect' users not also breastfeeding). This makes it somewhat like 'Implanon by mouth'.

Following a reassuring European study, in which Cerazette tablets were deliberately taken late, 12 hours of 'leeway' in pill-taking have been approved before extra precautions are advised – these then being for 2 days, as for other POPs (although the manufacturer's SPC still recommends 7 days). A major advantage of

Cerazette is its suitability for many young and highly fertile users for whom we would previously not even have suggested a POP. Realistically, despite recommended tricks such as setting one of their mobile phone alarms, busy or scatty individuals are sure to miss some POPs: but they are much more likely to get away with it on Cerazette.

Otherwise, Cerazette shares the medical safety and rapid reversibility – but also, unfortunately, the tendency to irregular bleeding side effects and functional ovarian cyst formation – of the old-type POPs.

Starting routines
See Table 9 (ie as other POPs). 'Missed pills' advice is on p.70.

Advantages and indications
- For a start, Cerazette is obviously free of all the risks attributable to EE; in addition, no effects on BP have been reported. Hence, it greatly broadens the indications for a progestogen-only method, in many cases where a COC is WHO 4 or 3, but a Pill method with greater efficacy than ordinary POPs is desired.
- Cerazette is now a good option for many young fertile women with complicated structural heart disease or pulmonary hypertension (see above); or undergoing major or leg surgery.
- Given the earlier discussion about POPs and *body mass*, Cerazette would now be the first-choice POP for a woman weighing over 70 kg, unless she was breastfeeding or over 45 years of age, in which case any POP in normal daily dose would be effective.
- Cerazette also usually ablates the menstrual cycle like COCs do, but without using EE. So it has potentially beneficial effects and can be tried (but not always successfully – no promises possible) in a range of disorders, including:
  - past history of ectopic pregnancy (discussed above)
  - dysmenorrhoea
  - menorrhagia
  - mittelschmerz
  - premenstrual syndrome (PMS).

Problems and disadvantages
As with all progestogen-only methods, irregular bleeding remains a very real problem. Indeed, this is the one area

showing no great advantage in the pre-marketing comparative study with LNG 30 μg POP-users. The dropout rate for changes in bleeding pattern showed no difference, but among those who persevered, there was a useful trend for the more annoying frequent and prolonged bleeding experiences to lessen with continued use.

Despite this higher incidence of (more acceptable) oligo-amenorrhoea than with existing POPs, Cerazette (like other POPs and Implanon) still appears to provide adequate follicular-phase levels of estradiol (see above).

Contraindications

These, whether WHO 4, 3 or 2, are very similar to those for old-type POPs. The main difference is that Cerazette is more effective, making it positively suitable for a past history of ectopic pregnancy.

In summary:

Cerazette may well become a first-line hormonal contraceptive for many women. However, there is no indication to use it rather than a cheaper old-type POP in lactation or in older women, especially in those above 45 years of age. One cannot expect to improve upon 100% contraception, which, in combination with an ordinary POP, these two states do (almost) provide!

Background

In the UK, the only injectable currently licensed for long-term use is depot medroxyprogesterone acetate (DMPA) – Depo-Provera – and it has been given additional approval as a first-line contraceptive. It has been repeatedly endorsed by the expert committees of prestigious bodies, such as the International Planned Parenthood Federation and WHO. DMPA is even safer than COCs, in spite of the adverse publicity it often receives.

Anxiety about this method was generated by animal research of very doubtful relevance to humans. WHO data indicate that DMPA-users have a reduced risk of cancer, with no overall increased risk of cancers of the breast, ovary or cervix – and a fivefold reduction in the risk of carcinoma of the endometrium (relative risk 0.2). There is still the possibility of a weak cofactor effect on breast cancer in young women similar to that with COCs. However, this is unproven, and the apparent association may be due to surveillance bias in early years of use by the younger women.

Administration

There are actually two injectable agents available: DMPA 150 mg every 12 weeks, and Noristerat (norethisterone enanthate; Schering Health Care) 200 mg every 8 weeks, both given by deep intramuscular injection in the first 5 days of the menstrual cycle. Injections may also be given beyond day 5, with 7 days added precautions if it is near certain that a conception risk has not been taken. The injection sites, in the UK usually in the right upper quadrant of either buttock, should not be massaged.

Noristerat is not licensed for long-term contraception, though it can be so used off-licence (p. 150),and will not be considered further here.

Subcutaneous DMPA

There is interest in this different route of administration, under the skin of the abdominal wall or upper thigh. The US-marketed product is termed depo-subQ provera 104. Not yet available in the UK, it delivers a lower dose of medroxyprogesterone acetate (104 mg) than standard Depo-Provera for a similar duration of effectiveness. Work is in progress to provide it in Uniject – a one-time-use injection system that is simple, foregoes vials and syringes, and is virtually impossible to re-use. Hopefully, this could also lead to the woman being given supplies annually for self-administration.

Mechanism of action and effectiveness

DMPA is one of the most effective among reversible methods (Table 1), with a 'perfect use' failure rate of 0.3% and a typical use failure rate of 3% in the first year of use. It functions primarily by causing anovulation, backed by similar effects on the cervical mucus to the COC, as back-up. A high initial blood level is achieved, declining over the next 3 months but staying above the level to inhibit ovulation for much longer in some women.

Potential drug interactions (Re lamotrigine, see p. 51)

Contrary to previous advice, since it has been shown that the liver ordinarily clears the blood reaching it completely of the drug – and enzyme-inducers obviously cannot increase clearance beyond 100% – there is no requirement to shorten the injection interval. This applies even to users of the most powerful enzyme-inducers, rifampicin or rifabutin.

> ### Starting routines – timing of the first injection
> - In *menstruating women*, the first injection should ideally be given on day 1, but can be up to day 5 of the cycle; if given later than day 5 (including *much* later if abstinence believably claimed to that day), advise 7 days' extra precautions.

- If a woman is *on a COC or POP or Cerazette* up to the day of injection, the injection can normally be given any time, with no added precautions.
- *Postpartum* (when the woman is not breastfeeding) or *after a second-trimester abortion*, the first injection should normally be at about day 21, and if later with added precautions for 7 days. If later and still amenorrhoeic, pregnancy risk must be excluded (p. 145). Earlier use can lead to prolonged heavy bleeding, but is sometimes clinically justified.
- During *lactation*, if chosen, DMPA is best given at 6 weeks. Lactation is *not* inhibited at all. The dose to the infant is small, and believed to be entirely harmless beyond 6 weeks.
- After *miscarriage* or a *first-trimester abortion:* injection on the day, or after expulsion of fetus if a medical procedure was used. If the injection is given beyond the 7th day, advise 7 days' extra precautions.

Overdue injections of DMPA with continuing sexual intercourse

WHOSPR permit injections to be up to 2 weeks late without the need for any additional method. This will very often be an effective strategy. However, as rare conceptions in the UK have been reported to the manufacturer as early as the end of the 13th week, I recommend a rather more cautious protocol, as in the following box:

Protocol for late injection, with continuing unprotected intercourse

- From day 85 to day 91 (13th week), give injection plus condoms or equivalent to be used during the next 7 days
- From day 92 to day 98 (14th week), give the injection, plus EC (usually by a hormone method) plus condoms for 7 days (no pregnancy testing):
- Beyond day 98 (end of 14th week), the next injection is best postponed, but usually not for long: if possible, agreement is reached with the woman that she will either abstain or use condoms with greater care than ever before, UNTIL there has been a total of 14 days since the last sexual exposure. If a sensitive (20–25 IU/l) pregnancy test is *then* negative, the chances of a conception are negligible, no EC would usually be needed; and
  - The next dose can be given plus the usual advice for 7 further days of added barrier contraception; and

---

- A follow-up pregnancy test in a further 2 weeks might be wise.
- If the woman is not prepared to abstain or use condoms for the necessary days to reach 14 since her last sex, a useful compromise is to provide the POP (e.g. Cerazette) for that time – and then proceed as above. The teratogenic risks to a fetus exposed to the POP have been established as very low.

In all circumstances, counsel the woman regarding possible failure and the need for a check pregnancy test if there is doubt.

What should NOT happen is the woman who is over 2 weeks late with her injection being told to go away until she has her next period!

Note: DMPA may always be given *early,* though this is not advisable sooner than 4 weeks after a previous dose.

Advantages and indications

DMPA has obvious contraceptive benefits (it is effective and 'forgettable'), but the data imply that it also shares most of the non-contraceptive benefits of the COC described above, including protection against pelvic infection and endometrial cancer.

Main indications
- The woman's desire for a highly effective method that is independent of intercourse and unaffected by enzyme inducers, and
- When other options are contraindicated or disliked.
- A past history of ectopic pregnancy or, like all other progestogen-only methods, of
- Thrombosis (see earlier comments for the POP) – e.g. for effective contraception while waiting for major or leg surgery (Cerazette is another option here).

Non-contraceptive indications
- endometriosis
- past symptomatic functional cysts
- sickle cell anaemia
- epilepsy, in which it often reduces the frequency of seizures.

Problems and disadvantages

Metabolic changes are minimal, except for some evidence of reduction in HDL cholesterol (DMPA is therefore not a good method in atherogenic states).

Main side-effects:
- Irregular, sometimes prolonged, bleeding
- Amenorrhoea and potential hypo-estrogenism
- Impossibility of reversal of the effect of a dose (for at least 3 months, sometimes longer). It is unfair not to mention this fact in advance
- Delayed return of fertility – also something to warn about (see below)
- Weight gain (the latter can be marked in some cases) – again, forewarn!
- Some concern regarding reduced bone density – which is probably exaggerated.

Menstrual abnormalities
These are an obstacle to any large increase in the method's popularity.

Management of frequent or prolonged bleeding
- First, check that it does not have a non-DMPA-related cause (e.g. *Chlamydia* – see p. 57).
- Advise that it has a better prognosis than with implants, usually being an early problem that is then generally followed by amenorrhoea after 3–6 months.
- If it does not resolve, the next injection may be given early (but not less than 4 weeks since the last dose). However:
- Clinical experience suggests that giving additional estrogen is more successful – though not proven in trials. The rationale is to provide estrogen cyclically to produce some 'physiological curettages', i.e. withdrawal bleeds designed to clear out the existing endometrium that is bleeding in an unacceptable way – in the hope that a 'better' endometrium and a more acceptable bleeding pattern will be obtained post treatment. The plan should be explained to the woman, who should also be pre-warned that it is unlikely to be so good as during the short-term COC.
- Possible treatments are:
  - EE 30 μg (as such, or more usually within a pill formulation such as Microgynon 30) given daily for 21 days, usually for 3 cycles. Courses may be repeated if an acceptable bleeding pattern does not follow. Or
  - if the woman has a WHO 4 contraindication to EE, one might try an alternative that was effective short term to stop bleeding with *Implanon* (see below), in a pilot study, namely doxycycline 100 mg bd for 5 days. The benefit is probably independent of an effect on Chlamydial endometritis, but test for this first.

Amenorrhoea occurs in most long-term users and is usually very acceptable, after the explanation if necessary that 'no blood is coming away because there IS no blood to come away', and moreover that 'menstruation has no excretory function or health benefits'.

Bone density and related issues

Does prolonged hypo-estrogenism in some women through use of DMPA (with or without oligo-amenorrhoea) lead, by analogy with premature menopause, to added risk of bone density loss or frank osteoporosis, or possibly arterial disease in those already predisposed, such as smokers?

Heart disease

A report regarding current DMPA use by the WHO in 1998 was reassuring, but more data are needed, focusing on any delayed effects in long-term users.

Bone mineral density

After more than 20 years of research but no randomized controlled trials or adequate comparative studies, there remains uncertainty – not about the variably low follicular-phase estradiol levels that are found in DMPA-users, but about their implications for bone health. We know that:

- Mean bone density is lower in DMPA users than in controls in cross-sectional comparisons, including among women above age 45.
- This finding is unconnected to the bleeding pattern (it may or may not occur in women experiencing either amenorrhoea or irregular bleeding).
- It increases again upon discontinuation (suggestive of a real effect – but also very reassuring for reversibility).
- From limited evidence, the bone mineral density in adolescent DMPA users is lower than controls using implants (or COCs). This has raised concern that normal *peak bone mass* that is fully developed by age 25 might not be achieved in users.

Yet:

- Long-term DMPA-using women examined after their menopause versus lifetime never-users have *not* been shown to differ in their bone densities, suggesting recovery of bone mass after stopping.

- An excess of limb or vertebral fractures has never been shown in long-term DMPA-users.

Based on the above, WHOMEC therefore simply states that DMPA is WHO 2 for adolescents and for women over age 45. American and UK drug regulators have been more cautious, however – see below.

How long to use DMPA, in the UK?

The CSM circular (18 November 2004) had one main recommendation, namely '*careful re-evaluation of risks and benefits in all those who wish to continue use for more than 2 years'. Clinically, in the UK,* the following is now advised:

Protocols for choice and duration of use of DMPA
If strong risk factors for osteoporosis already exist, namely:
- known osteoporosis or osteopenia
- long-term corticosteroid treatment
- secondary amenorrhoea, due to anorexia nervosa or marathon-running

then DMPA is WHO 4 – but the category could become WHO 3 if a bone scan shows no osteopenia, the risk factor has ceased, and the young woman is now obtaining either natural estrogen during normal cycling or EE through the COC.

- *Under age 19*, due to the above concern that it may prevent achievement of peak bone mass, WHOMEC classifies DMPA as WHO 2; and the UK advice of November 2004 is similar, namely to use it first-line 'but **only** after other methods have been discussed' and are unsuitable or unacceptable.
- *Above age 45*, DMPA is also WHO 2 (because of the possibility of incipient ovarian failure and as 'gentler' methods are available, such as the POP, which would be equally effective at this age).

For all other women:
- DMPA remains a highly effective, safe and 'forgettable' method, usable by almost any woman in the childbearing years.
- In the UK, it is now perceived as *very useful for fairly short-term use, after which switching to another long-term method such as an implant would be usual*.
- There should be a regular 'formal' 2-yearly discussion and reassessment of alternatives, but *without blood tests or any imaging. Such (e.g. bone density scanning) would only be appropriate if indicated for that particular woman on*

> **specific clinical grounds.** It is not a routine part of the protocol.
> - Many will therefore choose to switch from DMPA to another long-acting method (e.g. to Implanon, IUD or IUS) after 2–4–6–8 years, or above age 45 to a POP. However:
> - If the woman wishes to use DMPA for longer – even much longer – it is as always her right to decide to do so, on the 'informed user–chooser' basis, after counselling about the uncertainty.

Remember, when all is said and done, that DMPA is clearly safer than the EE-containing COC!

As it is recommended as an alternative in the protocol above, are there not similar bone density concerns with long-term Implanon?

There are not – the data are reassuring *so far*: in a non-randomized comparative study described below, after 2 years, bone densities remained similar among Implanon-users to those among copper IUD-users. By analogy, there are no worries yet on this account with Cerazette either – or with the LNG-IUS (below), whose amenorrhoeic action is anyway primarily at the end-organ level (the endometrium).

Contraindications

Absolute contraindications for DMPA
- Past *severe arterial* diseases, or current very high risk thereof (because of the above evidence about low estrogen levels coupled with reports of lowered HDL cholesterol)
- Current osteopenia or severe risk factor(s) for osteoporosis, including chronic corticosteroid treatment (>5 mg prednisolone/day)
- Any serious adverse effect of COCs not certainly related solely to the estrogen (e.g. liver adenoma or cancer -- although WHOMEC classifies these as WHO 3)
- Recent breast cancer not yet clearly in remission (see below)
- Acute porphyria, even if latent, no history of actual attack (progestogens as well as estrogens are believed capable of precipitating these, and the injection is not 'removable')
- Undiagnosed genital tract bleeding
- Actual or possible pregnancy
- Hypersensitivity to any component.

Relative contraindications for DMPA

(WHO 2 unless otherwise stated)

- According to degree, except as first bullet above, arterial disease risk is WHO 2. Familial hyperlipidaemia (UKMEC) and in my view longstanding DM (see p. 83, last 3 lines) are WHO 3. Other progestogen-only methods such as the POP are preferred
- Short-term steroid treatment, recovered anorexia nervosa with normal menstrual cycling (see above – these are usually WHO 3)
- Under 18 or over 45 years of age are WHO 2 with respect to the bones (see above)
- Active liver disease with abnormal liver function tests – caution required (WHO 3) – but WHO 2 with normal biochemistry
- Recent trophoblastic disease is WHO 3 (UKMEC) until hCG is undetectable in blood as well as urine, then WHO 1
- DMPA is usable in all non-acute porphyrias (WHO 2)
- Sex-steroid-dependent cancer, including breast cancer, in complete remission is WHO 3 (after 5 years according to WHOMEC). However, a POP or LNG-IUS would be preferable (lower dose, more reversible)
- Unacceptability despite reassurance of menstrual irregularities, especially cultural/religious taboos whether associated with bleeding or amenorrhoea
- Obesity, although further weight gain is not inevitable (see below)
- Past severe endogenous depression
- Planning a pregnancy in the near future (see below)
- Bleeding tendency. This is WHO 2 or 3 with respect to deep haematoma risk, minimized by extra care when injections are given. With the INR in the normal range (2–3) warfarin treatment is only WHO 2, and does *not* contraindicate Implanon (below) which is inserted so superficially.

Counselling

There are just four main practical points that must always be made to prospective users:

- The effects, whether wanted (contraceptive) or unwanted, are *not reversible for the duration of the injection*: this fact is unique among current contraceptives.
- Weight gain is probable due to increased appetite, so it is useful (and can really work) to advise a pre-emptive plan to start taking extra exercise as well as watching diet ... It

may help some women's decision-making, that those who are not already overweight put on less than those who are.

- Irregular, sometimes prolonged, *bleeding may be a problem*, but the outlook is good, as it is usually followed after a few months by *amenorrhoea, which is not a problem.*

- After the last dose, *conception is commonly delayed* with a median delay of 9 months, which is of course only 6 months after cessation of the method, but in some individuals it could be well over 1 year. A comparative study in Thailand showed that almost 95% of previously fertile users had conceived by 28 months after their last injection. So there is *no evidence of permanent infertility* caused by the drug. With respect to continuing post-DMPA amenorrhoea:
  - if conception **is not** wanted, alternative contraception must begin for about 13 weeks since the last injection
  - If conception **is** wanted, spontaneous ovulation can be anticipated in most cases: if not, refer for investigation/treatment at about 12 months after the last injection.

Follow-up

Aside from ensuring the injections take place at the correct intervals, follow-up is primarily advisory and supportive:

- Prolonged or too frequent bleeding is managed as already described.
- BP is normally checked initially, but there is absolutely no need for it to be taken before each dose, as studies fail to show any hypertensive effect. An annual check is reasonable as well-woman care.

Contraceptive implants

Implants contain a progestogen in a slow-release carrier, made either of dimethylsiloxane, as in Jadelle (not available in the UK) with two implants, or ethylene vinyl acetate (EVA), as in Implanon, a single rod (Figure 12).

They are excellent examples of long-acting reversible contraceptives (LARCs), with the ideal 'forgettable' default state, yet rapid reversibility.

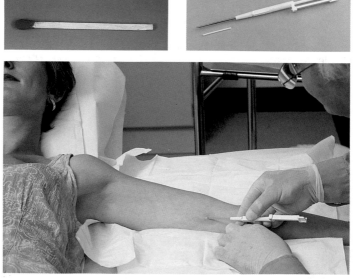

Figure 12
Implanon (courtesy of Organon Laboratories Ltd). Note that current advice is to insert anterior to the site shown (see text).

Mechanism of action, administration and effectiveness

Implanon works primarily by ovulation inhibition, supplemented mainly by the usual sperm-blocking mucus effect. It is a single 40 mm rod, just 2 mm in diameter, containing 68 mg of etonogestrel – the chief active metabolite of desogestrel – and so has much in common with Cerazette. This is dispersed in an EVA matrix and covered by a 0.06 mm rate-limiting EVA membrane.

Clinically:
- Implanon is inserted subdermally but very superficially under the skin over the biceps, medially in the upper arm, under local anaesthesia, from a dedicated sterile preloaded applicator by a simple injection-and-withdrawal technique – aided by the blunt bevel of its cleverly shaped wide-bore needle.
- Current teaching, contrary to the SPC, is to insert superficial to the biceps muscle and *anterior* to the groove between the triceps and biceps, well away from the neurovascular bundle.
- *Although this implant is much easier than Norplant to insert or remove, specific ('model arm' plus live) training is essential and cannot be obtained from any book.* In the UK, the best training is obtainable through the Faculty of FP. The manufacturer (Organon) can provide names of Faculty-approved trainers.
- After an initial phase of several weeks giving higher blood levels, Implanon delivers almost constant low daily levels of the hormone, for a recommended duration of use of 3 years.
- In the pre-marketing trials, Implanon had the unique distinction of a zero failure rate, although the 'perfect use' (= typical use) failure rate is now estimated as about 5 in 10 000 insertions.
- Nearly all 'failures' that have been reported either had had the insertion during a conception cycle or were failures to insert at all (hence the advice always to palpate the Implanon in situ just after insertion).
- *Effect of body mass:* in the international studies, serum levels tended to be lower in heavier women, but, given the high margin of efficacy, subsequently failures attributed to BMI have not occurred.
- Clinically, this finding should *not* detract in the slightest from offering Implanon to overweight women for whom the COC (or Evra) has a high VTE risk.
- *Earlier replacement?* The SPC says 'consider' this in the third year of use by 'heavier' women. Personally, I would only discuss this possibility in a young fertile woman with a BMI well over 100 kg if she began to cycle regularly in the third year (suggesting reliance only on the mucus effect).

Enzyme-inducer drug treatment

The SPC states that hepatic enzyme inducers may lower the blood levels of etonogestrel, but there have been no specific interaction studies. Therefore women on *short-term treatment* with any of these drugs are advised to use a barrier method in addition and (because reversal of enzyme induction always takes time) for 28 days thereafter. During *long-term enzyme-inducer drug treatment*, Organon recommends transfer to a non-hormonal method and removal of the Implanon. This seems a bit wasteful and may be resisted by satisfied users; moreover, those in monogamous relationships may reject the long-term use of barriers. So, despite the absence of specific trials, one might instead consider compensating for the enzyme induction by, for example, a daily Cerazette or even (expensively!) by a second Implanon. These prescriptions would be unlicensed and therefore used on a 'named-patient' basis (see p. 150).

However, since enzyme-inducer drug users do so well with DMPA or the LNG-IUS, these might be better as well as cheaper options, for long-term users. (Re lamotrigine, see p. 51.)

Reversibility and removal problems

Reversal is normally simple, with almost immediate effect. Under local anaesthesia, steady digital pressure on the proximal end of the Implanon with a 2 mm incision over the distal end leads to delivery of that end of the rod, removal being completed by grasping it with mosquito forceps. Again, removal *training* is crucial, using the 'model arm' and live under supervision. *Removal problems* can be minimized by good training, in both the insertion and removal techniques. *Difficult removals* correlate with initially too-deep insertion. Beware particularly of the thin or very muscular woman with very little subcutaneous tissue. Insertion can easily permit a segment of the rod to enter the (biceps) muscle, with deep migration following.

Specialized ultrasound techniques are required to localize 'lost' Implanons, and removal may need to be under ultrasound control: therefore Organon should be contacted for advice in all such cases.

Advantages and indications

The main indication is the woman's desire for a highly effective yet at all times rapidly reversible method, without the finality of sterilization, which is independent of intercourse: especially when other options are contraindicated or disliked.

- Above all, it provides efficacy and convenience: if the bleeding pattern suits, it is a 'forgettable' contraceptive.
- There is a long duration of action with one treatment (3 years), and high continuation rates.
- There is no initial peak dose given orally to the liver.
- Blood levels are low and steady, rather than fluctuating (as with the POP) or initially too high (as with injectables); this, with the previous point, means metabolic changes are minimal and negligible.
- Implanon is estrogen-free, and therefore definitely usable if there is a history of VTE (WHO 2).
- Median systolic and diastolic BP were unchanged in trials for up to 4 years.
- Being an anovulant, special indications include past ectopic pregnancy and as a possibility for menstrual disorders, although the outcome is not reliably beneficial (because of irregular bleeding – see below).
- The effects are rapidly reversible, an advantage over DMPA which is worth emphasising. After removal, serum etonogestrel levels were undetectable within one week, so return of fertility must be assumed to be almost immediate.

Disadvantages and contraindications

Local adverse effects may occur, namely:

- infection of the site
- expulsion
- migration and difficult removal (see above)
- scarring (very rare).

Contraindications are very similar to Cerazette since, like it but unlike DMPA, Implanon is an anovulant yet immediately reversible (and they contain essentially the same progestogen).

Absolute contraindications (WHO 4) for Implanon

- Any serious adverse effect of COCs not certainly related solely to the estrogen (e.g. liver adenoma or cancer: WHOMEC is more permissive, WHO 3)
- Recent breast cancer not yet clearly in remission (see below)
- Acute porphyria with history of actual attack precipitated by hormones; otherwise WHO 3
- Known or suspected pregnancy
- Undiagnosed genital tract bleeding
- Hypersensitivity to any component.

The manufacturer adds 'severe hepatic disease', which WHOMEC classifies as WHO 3, and 'active venous thromboembolic disorder', which presumably means a current episode – which is only WHO 2 according to UKMEC. There is no evidence that Implanon (like all other progestogen-only methods) can increase VTE risk.

Relative contraindications (WHO 3)

- Acute porphyria, latent, with no previous attack (use with forewarning/monitoring); Implanon is also usable in all the non-acute porphyrias
- Current severe liver disorder with persistent biochemical change
- Recent trophoblastic disease until hCG is undetectable in blood as well as urine; then WHO 1
- Sex-steroid-dependent cancer, including breast cancer, in complete remission (WHO advises 5 years). In all cases, agreement of the relevant hospital consultant should be obtained and the woman's autonomy respected: record that she understands it is unknown whether progestogen alone in Implanon alters the recurrence risk
- Enzyme-inducers – discussed above (but another method such as an DMPA, IUD or LNG-IUS would be preferable)
- Past symptomatic functional ovarian cysts – *might* recur using Implanon, especially in the third year.

Relative contraindications (WHO 2)

- Past VTE or severe risk factors for VTE; clinically, in fact, this is often an indication (see above)
- Risk factors for arterial disease; more than one risk factor can be present
- Current liver disorder, now with normal biochemistry
- Most other chronic severe systemic diseases
- Unacceptability of irregular menstrual bleeding – which remains a problem with all progestogen-only methods, certainly including Implanon.

Timing of Implanon insertion

- **In the woman's natural cycle**, day 1–5 is usual timing; if any later than day 5 (assuming no sexual exposure up to that day), recommend additional contraception for 7 days.
- If a woman is on COC or POP/Cerazette or DMPA, the implant can normally be inserted at any time, with no added precautions.

Clinical implications

Insertions only during the above tiny natural-cycle window are a logistic and conception risk nightmare! So a useful practice tip is actively to recommend use of an anovulant method (i.e. one of those in the second point, in the above box) at counselling, for use until the Implanon insertion. If the COC is chosen, it may usefully be run on ('tricycled'), so the implant is placed during already-established amenorrhoea

---

Timing in non-cycling states
- Following delivery (not breastfeeding) or second-trimester abortion, insertion on about day 21 is recommended, or if later with additional contraception for 7 days. If later and still amenorrhoeic, pregnancy risk should be excluded.
- If breastfeeding, insert on day 21–28 (UKMEC), with no need for added contraception for 7 days.
- Following first-trimester abortion, immediate insertion is best:
  - on the day of surgically induced abortion or the second part of a medical abortion, or
  - up to 7 days later
  - if >7 days later, an added method such as condoms is recommended for 7 days.

Counselling and ongoing supervision

Explain the likely changes to the bleeding pattern and the possibility of 'hormonal' side effects (see below). This discussion should as always be backed by a good leaflet, such as the FPA one, and well-documented.

No treatment-specific follow-up is necessary (including no need for BP checks). The SPC recommends one follow-up visit at 3 months. More important is an explicit 'open-house' policy, so the woman knows she can return at any time to discuss possible side effects, without any provider pressure to persevere if the woman really wants the implant removed (the standard for the maximum wait for removal should be no more than 2 weeks).

Bleeding problems

In the pre-marketing randomized controlled trial comparing Implanon with the old six-implant Norplant, the bleeding patterns were very similar:

- Amenorrhoea was significantly more common, as expected for an anovulant method.
- The infrequent bleeding and spotting rate (normally an acceptable pattern) was about 26%.
- Normal cycling was reported by 35% of women.
- However, the combined rates for the more annoying 'frequent bleeding and spotting' and 'prolonged bleeding and spotting' totalled 18% with Implanon.

Clinical management

With reassurance, most women are happy to accept one of the patterns in the first three points above. For the fourth group, perseverance beyond 3 months is rewarded less often than with DMPA. After eliminating unrelated causes for the bleeding (p. 57):

- The best short-term treatment is cyclical estrogen therapy to produce some 'pharmacological curettages' (i.e. withdrawal bleeds), on a similar basis to the above regimen for DMPA. This may most easily be provided by three cycles of Mercilon or Marvelon, after which the bleeding may (or sometimes may not!) become acceptable. As above, the plan should be explained to the woman, who should also understand that it is not certain to work. Courses may be repeated if an acceptable bleeding pattern does not follow. Or,
- If the woman has a WHO 4 contraindication to EE, an alternative that was effective short term in a pilot study is doxycycline 100 mg bd for 5 days. The mechanism is believed to be an effect on endometrial enzymes and is probably independent of treating any Chlamydial endometritis. But one should test for Chlamydia first, as usual with irregular bleeding.

Minor side-effects

Reported in frequency order, minor side-effects were:

- Acne (but this also sometimes improved!)
- Headache
- Abdominal pain
- Breast pain
- 'Dizziness'
- Mood changes (depression, emotional lability)
- Libido decrease
- Hair loss.

Weight gain

In the pre-marketing randomized controlled trial, the mean body weight increase over 2 years was 2.6% with Implanon and 2.9% with Norplant, while in a parallel study, similar users of an IUD showed weight increases of 2.4% in the same timescale. Weight seems to be less of a problem than with DMPA, although some individuals do find their weight gain unacceptable.

Bone mineral density

Since Implanon suppresses ovulation and does not supply any estrogen, the same questions as with DMPA arise over possible hypo-estrogenism However, it appears that, like Cerazette and other POPs, the suppression of FSH levels with Implanon is less complete, allowing higher follicular estrogen levels.

In a non-randomized comparative study, no bone density changes or differences in the means, ranges or standard errors were detected between 44 users of Implanon-users and 29 users of copper IUDs over 2 years, which is reassuring.

Intrauterine contraception

Intrauterine contraceptives are currently of two distinct types:

- copper intrauterine devices (IUDs), in which the copper ion (the actual contraceptive) is released from a band or wire on a plastic carrier
- the levonorgestrel-releasing intrauterine system, which releases that progestogen – this will be abbreviated below as either LNG-IUS or just IUS.

COPPER-BEARING DEVICES
'It is time to pardon the intrauterine device!'

This headline to an article says it all. Actually, there are 150 million users worldwide, but the lion's share is in just one country – China. It seems improbable that the difference between less than 1% of sexually active users in USA or 5% in the UK but 20% in France is explicable by some important difference between the French, the British and the US uterus. Do the Chinese and the French have something to teach the rest of the world?

In many countries, women in their late 30s have not been requesting IUDs because they were told in their 20s to avoid that method. This is strange, because in reality a woman in her later reproductive years with, say, two or three children, is the ideal user. The devices have changed somewhat, but more importantly she has too – a parous cervical canal makes insertion easier and commonly she also has less exposure to STIs than in her youth.

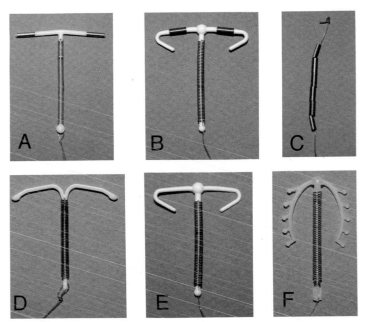

Figure 13
Copper IUDs. A: T-Safe Cu 380 A QL (Quick-Load) (FP Sales) or TT 380 Slimline (Durbin); B: Flexi-T 380 (FP Sales); C: GyneFix (Durbin, FP Sales); D: Nova-T 380 (Schering); also UT 380 Short (Durbin) with short stem; E: Flexi-T 300 (FP Sales) with short stem; F: Multiload Cu375 (Organon) or Load 375 (Durbin). (Reproduced by kind permission of Dr Anne MacGregor.)

Some doctors are complying too readily with requests for male or female sterilization that originate partly from 'medical myths' about the intrauterine alternative. Leaving aside the significant advance represented by the LNG-IUS, too few women know that the latest **banded copper IUDs** (Figure 13) are, in practice, comparable to reversible sterilization.

Advantages of copper IUDs – a long list!

- Safe: mortality 1:500 000
- Effective:
  - Immediately
  - Postcoitally (although this is not true of the LNG-IUS)

- Highly, like sterilization if one of the many clones of the T-Safe Cu 380A is used (see below)
- No link with coitus
- No tablets to remember
- Continuation rates are high and permitted duration of use can exceed 10 years
- Reversible – and there is evidence that this is true even when IUDs have been removed for one of the recognized complications.

Mechanism of action

- Appropriate studies indicate that copper IUDs operate primarily by preventing fertilization, the copper ion being toxic to sperm.
- Their effectiveness when put in postcoitally shows that they act additionally to block implantation. However, when IUDs are in situ long term, this seems to be a rarely needed secondary or back-up mechanism.

Clinical implication
- As in any given cycle this type of IUD might be working through the block of implantation, there is a small risk of 'iatrogenic' conception if a device is removed after mid-cycle, even if abstinence follows.
- Ideally, therefore, women should either use another method additionally from 7 days before planned device removal or, if this has not been the case, postpone removal until the next menses.
- If a device *must* be removed earlier, hormonal postcoital contraception may be indicated.

Choice of devices and effectiveness

In the UK, the 'gold standard' among IUDs for a parous woman without menstrual problems (if these are present, a LNG-IUS would be preferable) is any banded copper IUD (Figure 13). The devices available are: T-Safe Cu 380A or new variants with their copper bands sunk into the arms of the plastic frame, which are branded as TT 380 'Slimline' or T-Safe Cu 380A QL 'Quick Load' (these are available, respectively, from Durbin and FP Sales – see MIMS). The last two both have a simpler loading system than the fiddly plastic 'hat' of the older T-Safe Cu 380A.

In Sivin's Population Council randomized controlled trial this banded IUD type had statistically similar efficacy to the LNG-IUS. The cumulative failure rate of the CuT 380Ag to 10 years was only 1.4 per 100 women (compare a mean rate of 1.8 per 100 women at 10 years after female sterilization in the American CREST study from 1996). There were no failures at all after year 5!

Important influence of age on effectiveness

Copper IUDs are much more effective in the older woman – largely because of declining fertility. Over the age of 30, there is also a reduction in rates of expulsion and of PID – the latter is believed not to be the result of the older uterus resisting infection but rather because the older woman is generally less exposed to risk of infection (whether through her own lifestyle or that of her only partner).

Advantages of one of the banded IUDs

The efficacy of the T-Safe Cu 380A in one randomized controlled trial was greater than that of the alternative Nova T 380. It is licensed for 10 years and the data support effectiveness until *12 years* (even when fitted below age 40, see below). But the main advantage lies in the infrequency of re-insertions. Research in the past 50 years has so clearly shown the truth of both parts of the following slogan:

IUD Slogan 1
Insertion can be a factor in the causation of almost every category of IUD problems *and must fully related* problems become less common with increasing duration of use; therefore, why ever use a 5-year device when a 10-year one will fit?

What if the woman is nulliparous?

Note that nulliparity per se is *not* WHO 4 for this method! In a mutually monogamous relationship (especially above age 35), it should be seen as only WHO 2 for the IUD method. The T-Safe Cu 380A, and its clones the 'Slimline' and 'Quick Load', usually pass through the cervical canal surprisingly easily, in all parities. So they remain the first-choice devices even for nulliparae – although a smaller IUD (see the options below) may sometimes be unavoidable, for a comfortable and satisfactory fitting.

When to use other IUDs (e.g. Nova T380)
(Figure 13)

> **For emergency contraception (EC)**
> The Nova T 380 might be appropriate for a nulliparous woman *using it for EC* and planning (see p. 128) to have the device removed later, once established on a new method (such as say DMPA). Another good EC option for nulliparae is the Flexi-T 300, which is exceptionally small and has an easy push-in fitting technique with no separate plunger. But it has been reported to have a fairly high expulsion rate.

> **Difficult fittings**
> - *For long-term use*, the **Nova T 380** and the **UT 380 Short** (Nova T style but on a shorter stem, from Durbin) should usually be reserved for when the T-Safe Cu 380A or equivalent cannot be fitted, for some reason. The reason could be an unusually tight cervix or acute flexion of the uterus – rare in parous women but not uncommon in nulliparae.
> - There is now also available the **Flexi-T 380,** on a slightly larger frame and with bands on its sidearms but otherwise identical in shape. We need more data on this – sought but not so far forthcoming! It *might* be very effective and usable for longer than its 5-year licensed life, be as easily inserted as the Flexi-T 300, and have an acceptable expulsion rate. If all that were true, in difficult cases, being copper-banded, it *might* come to rival the T-Safe Cu 380A and its clones, above. At present, we lack the data to be sure.
> - The **Multiload IUDs**, even the 375 thicker wire versions, were – in most of the randomized controlled trials – generally significantly less effective than the T-Safe Cu 380A, *with no firm evidence of the reputed better expulsion rate.*

When to use the banded but frameless GyneFix? (Figure 13)

This unique frameless device features a knot that is embedded by its special inserter system in the fundal myometrium. Below the knot, its polypropylene thread bears six copper bands and locates them within the uterine cavity. Being frameless, it is less likely to cause uterine pain, and when correctly inserted it appears to rival the efficacy of the T-Safe Cu 380A. Unfortunately, in routine UK practice it was found to have a high (rather than the expected low) expulsion rate – and all users should be forewarned about the risk of *unrecognized* expulsion. Being able to feel the threads is particularly important with GyneFix.

If it is available (by referral to someone trained in the specific insertion skills required), **indications for GyneFix** include:
- Distorted cavity on ultrasound scan (if IUD useable at all)
- A small uterine cavity sounding <6 cm (rival and probably more available options if uterus sounds to be at least 5 cm are the (banded) **Flexi-T 380™ or the (wire) Flexi-T 300 and UT 380 Short**)
- Previous history of expulsion or removal of a framed device that was accompanied by excessive cramping, within hours or days of insertion.

Aren't the names of copper IUDs confusing?

Fortunately, from now onwards, all mentions of either 'IUD' or 'copper IUD' will refer, unless otherwise stated, only to the **T-Safe Cu 380A** or one of its easy-loading variants.

Main problems and disadvantages of copper IUDs

The main medical problems are listed in the following box and dealt with in more detail thereafter. This is actually a remarkably short list as compared with hormonal methods.

Possible problems with copper IUDs
1. Intrauterine pregnancy – hence its risk, including miscarriage
2. Extrauterine pregnancy – as this is prevented less well than intrauterine (although the absolute risk is actually reduced in population terms)
3. Expulsion – hence the risks of pregnancy/miscarriage
4. Perforation, with:
   - risks to bowel/bladder and again
   - risks of pregnancy
5. Pelvic infection – as with (2), the IUD is *not* causative
6. Malpositioning – which predisposes to (1), (3) and (7)
7. Pain
8. Bleeding:
   - increased amount
   - increased duration.

Note, clinically from above that:

IUD Slogan 2
Pain and bleeding in IUD-users might signify a potentially dangerous condition – until proved otherwise.

This means that all of the first six problems need to be excluded as diagnoses before pain and bleeding are ascribed simply to being side effects of this method.

In situ conception

If the woman wishes to go on to full-term pregnancy, after a pelvic ultrasound scan, *the device should normally be removed*. This is counter-intuitive, because one would think that it would increase the miscarriage rate. The truth is the reverse: for example, with in situ failures of the Copper T 200 device, the normal rate of spontaneous abortion was 55%, dropping to 20% if the device was removed. The woman should of course be warned that an increased risk of miscarriage still remains.

Other clinical points:
- If the woman is going to have a termination of her pregnancy, her IUD (or IUS) can be removed at the planned surgery; however, it is safest to remove it before any medical abortion.
- If the threads are already missing when she is seen and other causes are excluded, aided by an ultrasound scan (see below): *the pregnancy is at increased risk of*:
  - second-trimester abortion (which could be infected)
  - antepartum haemorrhage
  - premature labour.
- If the woman goes on to full term, it is essential to identify clearly the device in the products of conception. If it is not found, a postpartum X-ray should be arranged in case the device is embedded or malpositioned or has perforated. There have been medicolegal cases when this was not done, because of an undiagnosed perforation; or because of unnecessary tests and treatments for 'infertility' when trying for a later wanted pregnancy, caused by a much earlier malpositioned IUD with no visible threads remaining in situ, ever since the original delivery.

There is no evidence of associated **teratogenicity** with conception during or immediately after use of copper devices.

IUDs with 'lost threads'

This symptom of 'lost threads' links together points (1), (3) and (4) in the box on p. 105. There are at least six causes of this condition – three with and three without pregnancy. An intra-abdominal IUD is just as useless at stopping pregnancy as one that has been totally expelled. More commonly the woman is already pregnant and the threads have been drawn up or the device has altered its position in situ.

IUD Slogan 3

The woman with 'lost threads' is already pregnant until proven otherwise – moreover, even then, she is likely to be unprotected and at risk of becoming pregnant.

'**Lost threads' – six possible causes**

Pregnant	Not pregnant
Unrecognized expulsion + pregnancy	Unrecognized expulsion + not yet pregnant
Perforation + pregnancy	Perforation + not yet pregnant
Device in situ + pregnancy	Device in situ + malpositioned or threads short (in uterus, if not found in cervical canal)

Diagnosis and management may involve some or all of the examinations and techniques shown in Figure 14. In this flow diagram, the later stages should follow referral to a specialist.

More about perforation

This has a general estimated risk for all IUDs of about 1 per 1000 insertions, but the exact rate (as for expulsion) depends much less on the IUD design than on the skill of the clinician. Perforated devices should now almost always be removable at laparoscopy.

Pelvic inflammatory disease and IUDs – What is the truth?

This is the great fear we all have about IUDs. Just as the Pill has been blamed for problems that we now know were due to smoking, copper IUDs have been blamed for infections that were really acquired sexually (see the Chinese evidence, below).

Much of the anxiety derived from the Dalkon Shield disaster – but this was a unique device with a polyfilamentous thread, facilitating the transfer by capillary action of potential pathogens from the lower to the upper genital tract. Modern copper devices have a monofilamentous thread. They do not themselves cause infection. However, they provide no protection against PID (in

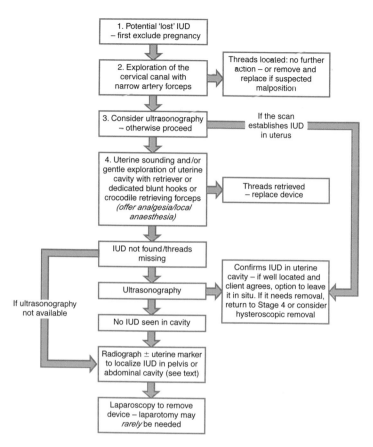

Figure 14
Management of 'lost' IUD threads.

contrast to the LNG-IUS: see below), and there is some suspicion that the infections that occur may perhaps be more severe as a result of the foreign-body effect.

In a classic WHO study, Farley et al (*Lancet* 1992; **339**: 785–8) reported on a database from a number of WHO randomized controlled trials, including approximately 23 000 insertions worldwide – and in every country *but one*, the same pattern emerged (Figure 15):

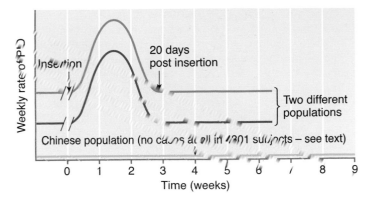

Figure 15
WHO study of 22,900 IUD insertions (4301 in China) in Europe, Africa, Asia and the Americas. Note that the weekly rate of pelvic inflammatory disease (PID) returns to the preinsertion background rate for the population studied.

- There was an IUD-associated increased risk of infection for 20 days after the insertion.
- However, the weekly infection rate 3 weeks after insertion went back to the same weekly rate as existed before insertion, i.e. the norm for that particular society.

In China, the one exception, there were no infections diagnosed at all in spite of 4301 insertions. In another two studies from China also done in the 1980s, a further 3300 IUD-users were followed for over a year, again with no cases of PID

Interpretation
These findings are interpreted as follows:

- The post-insertion infection 'hump' of infections cannot the result of a bad insertion technique, restricted to doctors outside China.
- It is much more likely that, although the doctors in all th centres were searching for truly monogamous couples, they were only successful in this search in China (durin the 1980s, when it is well recognised that China was practically an STI-free zone – China is no longer unique this respect today).

- In the other countries, PID-causing organisms (especially *Chlamydia trachomatis*) are presumed to have been present – no cervical prescreening being available at that time – in a proportion of the women. The process of insertion would interfere with natural defensive mechanisms (as has been confirmed when there is instrumentation in other contexts, such as therapeutic abortion).
- This would enable organisms to spread from the lower genital tract, where they had previously resided asymptomatically, into the upper genital tract, so causing the PID.

In summary, therefore:

IUD Slogan 4
IUDs, intrinsically, cannot be the cause of the PID that occurs in IUD users. Otherwise, how could there have been so many as 7600 Chinese users in the 1980s and not a single attack?!

- The greatest risk is in the first 20 days, most probably caused by pre-existing carriage of sexually transmitted infections.
- Risk thereafter, as with pre-insertion, relates to the background risk of STIs (high in Africa, but so low in mainland China in the 1980s that it seems to have been absent in the study population).

Therefore, the *evidence-based policy* should be that:
- Elective IUD insertions and reinsertions should always occur through a 'Chinese cervix', i.e. one that has been established to be pathogen-free, so hopefully eliminating the post-insertion infections shown in Figure 15.

Clinical implications for IUD insertion arrangements
- Prospective IUD users should always be verbally screened, meaning a good sexual history (p. 6). They need to know that they will need to use condoms too if the method is judged WHO 3 because of situational high STI risk – or even abandon this choice and use another method altogether (WHO 4).
- 'When did you last have sex with someone different?' means a rethink about the IUD method if that was within the past 3 months.

- Also – and this is the thorny one we all tend to leave out – 'Do you ever wonder if your partner has or is likely to have another sexual relationship?' (*Reworded as appropriate, and always with the utmost tact.*)
- In populations with high prevalence of *C. trachomatis* (say >5% incidence – and note it is around twice that in most recent UK surveys of the under-25s), this verbal screen should be backed by modern DNA-based (ligase chain reaction (LCR) or polymerase chain reaction (PCR)) *Chlamydia* prescreening. This is as important for reinsertions as for initial IUD insertions.
- Recent exposure history or evidence of a purulent discharge from the cervix indicates referral for more detailed investigation at a genitourinary medicine (GUM) clinic. If *Chlamydia* is detected, the woman should be referred to a GUM service:
  - to be investigated for linked pathogens
  - to have necessary treatment and contact tracing arranged
  - and *usually* have the IUD insertion postponed.
- *In emergency contraception cases*, screen – but treat anyway before the result is available (e.g. with azithromycin 1 g stat).
- The cervix should be cleansed very thoroughly (primarily physically, by swabbing) before any device is inserted, with minimum trauma, following the manufacturer's instructions.
- In addition to the routine 6-week follow-up visit, the woman should be given clear details of the relevant symptoms of PID, and instructed as routine to telephone the practice nurse about 1 week post-insertion. This should identify any women with an early infection (during the crucial 20 post-insertion days of Figure 11).

The *Chlamydia* screen can of course be omitted if, for example, the woman is over 35 years of age *and* the sexual history of 'mutual' monogamy is strong, particularly if her family is considered complete.

'Blind' prescription of an appropriate antibiotic is necessary in emergency cases, but the screening should still be done. Otherwise contact tracing is impossible and re-infection will simply occur later, the woman becoming one of the regular weekly cases that happen later than the first 20 days (Figure 15).

Actinomyces-like organisms (ALOs)
These are sometimes reported in cervical smears – more commonly with long duration of use of either IUDs or IUSs.

If ALOs are reported:

Plan A. First, call the woman for an extra consultation and examination, particularly bimanually. If all is normal, see below. But:
- If there are relevant symptoms or signs (pain, dyspareunia, excessive discharge, tenderness or any suggestion of an adnexal mass) then an ultrasound scan should then be arranged, with a low threshold for gynaecological referral.
- After preliminary discussion with the microbiologist, the device should be removed and sent for culture. Treatment will have to be vigorous, usually prolonged, if frank pelvic actinomycosis is actually confirmed – it is a potentially life-threatening and fertility-destroying condition, although very rare.

Much more usually, the ALO finding occurs in asymptomatic and physical-sign-free women – who stay that way. Over-reaction might cause more morbidity, through pregnancy, than through actinomycosis, given the latter's rarity.

Second part of protocol on detection of ALOs
When there are no positive clinical findings, in consultation with the woman, the clinician may decide between **either of the following approaches, B or C:**

Plan B
- Simple removal with or without reinsertion, and without antibiotic treatment.
- Advise the woman, along with written reference material, about the relevant symptoms that should make her seek a doctor urgently and tell them that she recently had an IUD or IUS plus ALOs.
- Repeat a cervical smear after 3 months (it will nearly always be negative) with a re-check bimanual examination. Both smear-taking and IUD follow-up then revert to normal.

Plan C
- Leave the IUD or IUS alone after the initial thorough and fully reassuring examination, preferably backed by a negative pelvic ultrasound scan.
- Advise the woman, and provide her with written material, about the relevant symptoms that should make her seek a doctor urgently and tell them that she has been followed up with an IUD or IUS plus ALOs.
- Arrange meticulous follow-up, initially at 6 months, including a check for symptoms and bimanual examination.

Given the data that device removal usually clears the ALO finding, even though long-term use is normally best, there is much to be said for following plan A+B rather than A+C as above. In either case, keep a good-quality record of the consultation.

Is ectopic pregnancy caused by copper IUDs?

This is another myth. The main cause of ectopics is previous tubal infection, with one or both tubes being damaged. The non-causative association with IUDs comes about because they are *even more* effective at preventing pregnancy *in the uterus than in the tube*.

Ectopic pregnancies are actually reduced in number, because very few sperm get through the copper-containing uterine fluids to reach an egg, so very few implantations can occur in any damaged tube. However, there are even fewer implantations in the uterus. Thus, in the ratio of ectopic/intrauterine pregnancies, the denominator is reduced more than the numerator. So ectopics are more likely among IUD-pregnancies – even though both types of pregnancy are actually reduced in frequency.

The estimated rate of ectopic pregnancy for sexually active Swedish women seeking pregnancy is 1.2–1.6 per 100 woman-years. The risk in users of either the T-Safe Cu 380A and its clones or of the LNG-IUS is estimated as 0.02 per 100 woman-years, which is at least 60 times lower.

Accordingly, UKMEC classifies a past history of ectopic pregnancy as WHO 1. *Clinically,* however, some caution is still necessary:

IUD Slogan 5
Any IUD-user with pain and a late period or irregular bleeding has an ectopic pregnancy until proved otherwise.

Moreover, since there are even better anovulant options (e.g. COC, Cerazette, or DMPA), for nulliparae I continue to view a past history of ectopic pregnancy as a relative contraindication (WHO 3) to IUDs. See p. 119.

Pain and bleeding

As already stated in IUD Slogan 1 (p. 101), pain and bleeding in IUD-users signify a dangerous condition – until proved otherwise.

As well as excluding conditions such as infection or an ectopic pregnancy or miscarriage, consider malpositioning of the frame of an IUD, which can cause pain through uterine spasms. Indeed, beyond the first few post-insertion days, a well-located IUD or IUS rarely causes pain.

Copper devices do increase:
- the *duration* of bleeding by a mean of 1–2 days
- the measured *volume* of bleeding by about one-third (although this can be a hardly noticeable addition if the woman's normal periods are light)
- in a population of users of copper-IUDs, haemoglobin levels tend to fall, in contrast to LNG-IUD users, and some with losses above 80 ml/cycle are prone to frank anaemia.

Bleeding problems usually settle with time. If they do not, it may be necessary to change the method of contraception – perhaps to the LNG-IUS (see below).

Drug treatments may reduce the loss, but are not very satisfactory in the long term. The most successful therapies are mefenamic acid 500 mg 8-hourly (which can simultaneously help pain as well, and so is usually tried first) and tranexamic acid 1–1.5 g 8-hourly.

Duration of use

Studies regularly show *reduced* rates of discontinuation with increasing duration of use – whether for expulsion, infection or pain and bleeding, or indeed pregnancy. Coupled with the fact that most IUD complications are insertion-related, it is good news that the banded devices T-Safe Cu 380A and clones may be used for 10 years or longer.

Above the age of 40, the agreed policy, since a 1990 statement in the *Lancet* by the FPA and the predecessor body of the Faculty of FP, is as follows:

IUD Slogan 6

Any copper device (even a copper-wire-only type) that has been fitted above the age of 40 may be used for the rest of reproductive life.

It never needs replacement, even though not licensed for that long. For the duration of use of the LNG-IUS in various situations, see below.

Cancer risk

After much work, both in animals or humans, the development of cancer in the uterus of long-term users has never been identified as a risk from either copper IUDs or of the LNG-IUS discussed below. Indeed, there is a hint from the research, even with copper IUDs, of a reduced risk of endometrial carcinoma.

THE LEVONORGESTREL-RELEASING INTRAUTERINE SYSTEM

A schematic of the LNG-IUS (Mirena, Schering Health Care) is shown in Figure 16.

Method of action and effectiveness

Main features of the LNG-IUS

- It releases about 20 μg/24 hours of LNG from its polydimethyl-siloxane reservoir, through a rate-limiting membrane, for its licensed 5 years (and longer).
- Its main contraceptive effects are local, through changes to the cervical mucus and uterotubal fluid that impair sperm migration, backed by endometrial changes impeding implantation.
- Its cumulative failure rate to 7 years was very low, at 1.1 per 100 women in the large Sivin study – even less to 5 years in a European multicentre trial by Anderson et al.
- Its efficacy is not detectably impaired by enzyme-inducing drugs.
- The systemic blood levels of LNG are under half of the mean levels in users of the LNG POP (for users, this can be explained as 'like taking three old-type POPs per week'), and so although ovarian function is altered in some women, especially in the first year, 85% show the ultrasound changes of normal ovulation.
- The amount of LNG in the blood is still enough to give unwanted hormone-type side effects in some women; otherwise, irregular light bleeding is the main problem.
- Even if they become amenorrhoeic – as many do, primarily through a local end-organ effect – in those who do not ovulate (as well as the majority who do), sufficient estrogen is produced for bone health.
- Return of fertility after removal is rapid, and appears to be complete.

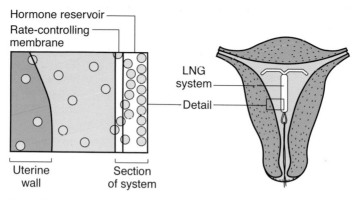

Figure 16
The levonorgestrel-releasing intrauterine system (LNG-IUS).

Advantages and indications

The user of this method can expect the following advantages:

- A dramatic reduction in amount and, *after the first few months* (discussed below), duration of blood loss.
- Dysmenorrhoea is improved in most women, and (for unexplained reasons) so are the symptoms of PMS in some.
- The LNG-IUS is the contraceptive method of choice for most women with menorrhagia and it prevents/treats iron-deficiency anaemia. Indeed it should still be a first-line treatment when contraception is not needed, for both menorrhagia and for menstrual pain (the latter even with normal blood loss).
- Endometriosis: gynaecologists now recognise the LNG-IUS as often ideal for long-term maintenance therapy, after initial diagnosis and treatment.
- Hormone-replacement therapy (HRT): by providing progestogenic protection of the uterus during estrogen replacement by any chosen route, the LNG-IUS uniquely, before final ovarian failure, offers 'forgettable, contraceptive, no-period and no PMS-type HRT'. For this increasingly popular indication, the LNG-IUS is currently licensed for 4 years before it must be replaced.
- Epilepsy: in a small series at the MPC, this was a very successful method for this condition, even in women on enzyme-inducer treatment.
- The LNG-IUS is, in short, a highly convenient and 'forgettable' contraceptive – with added gynaecological value.

The *contraceptive* advantages shown in the box above are, of course, shared with the T-Safe Cu 380A, which is the current gold standard for copper IUDs. However, this is where the similarity ends. The LNG-IUS fundamentally 'rewrites the textbooks' about IUDs, really only sharing the intrauterine location and certainly deserving a separate category (hence 'IUS').

What about infection/ectopic pregnancy risk and risk to future fertility?

Although IUDs do not themselves cause PID (see above), they fail to prevent it, and there is a suspicion that they sometimes worsen the attacks that occur. The LNG-IUS may actually reduce the frequency of clinical PID, perhaps through the progestogenic effect on cervical mucus, particularly in the youngest age groups who are most at risk. *However,* the risk is certainly not eliminated and condom use should still be advocated. But the available data make it possible to offer the LNG-IUS to some young women requesting a 'forgettable' contraceptive who would not be good candidates for conventional copper IUDs. Their future fertility is most unlikely to be adversely affected.

The data published for this device show (like the banded copper IUDs) a massive *reduction in ectopic risk,* which can be attributed to its greater efficacy by the sperm-blocking mechanism that reduces the risk of pregnancy in any site. However, in the case of a past history of an ectopic pregnancy, an anovulant method would be *even better.*

Problems and disadvantages of the LNG-IUS

As with any intrauterine device:
- *Expulsion* can occur, and there is the usual small risk of:
- *Perforation*, minimized by its 'withdrawal' as opposed to a 'plunger' technique of insertion.
- *Pain*, which suggests malpositioning as unexpected, pain is usually *improved* with an IUS. Check by ultrasound scan, indeed ahead of insertion whenever fibroids are suspected at the preliminary examination.
- A significant problem is the high incidence in the first post-insertion months of *uterine bleeding*, which, although small in quantity, may be very frequent or continuous and can cause considerable inconvenience. In later months:
- *Amenorrhoea* is commonly reported – sometimes *perceived* as a problem.

For both of these last two problems, particularly the former, 'forewarned is forearmed', through good counselling.

Women can accept the early weeks of light bleeding, even if very frequent, as a worthwhile price to pay for all the other advantages of the method: provided they are well informed in advance of LNG-IUS fitting. They can be confident that perseverance will be rewarded, since this early problem has such a good prognosis. The oligo-amenorrhoea that follows can be explained and interpreted to a woman as an advantage – gently debunking the myth that menstruation serves an excretory function – *not* an adverse side effect but a positive benefit of the method.

Women should also be forewarned that, although this method is mainly local in its action, it is not exclusively so. Therefore there is a small incidence of *'hormonal' side-effects* such as bloatedness, acne and depression. These do usually improve, often within 2 months, in parallel with the known decline in the higher initial LNG blood levels.

Functional ovarian cysts are also more common, although they are usually asymptomatic. If pain results, they should be investigated/monitored, but they usually resolve spontaneously.

Contraindications

Many of the contraindications of this method are shared with copper IUDs (see below). The additional few that are unique to LNG-IUS, due to the actions of its LNG hormone, are discussed in the following box. The manufacturer tends to be more cautious in calling them all WHO 4.

Unique contraindications (mainly WHO 3) for the LNG-IUS
- Current liver tumour or severe active hepatocellular disease
- Current severe active arterial or venous thrombotic disease (the former is WHO 2 according to UKMEC)
- Current breast cancer – this is WHO 4 according to UKMEC, with the LNG-IUS becoming usable on a WHO 3 basis after 5 years' remission, like all the other progestogen-only methods. In my view:
  - since the LNG-IUS gives the lowest systemic hormone dose of such methods, and
  - given the suggestive data that it may protect against tamoxifen-induced pre-cancer changes in the endometrium, in

---

selected cases this WHO 3 status might be agreed consider-
ably sooner, after consultation with the oncologist
- Trophoblastic disease (any) – this is WHO 3 while blood hCG
levels are high, as for other progestogen-only methods
(UKMEC), *but* there is no problem (WHO 1) after full recovery
- Hypersensitivity to levonorgestrel or other constituent (WHO 4).

In addition, *the LNG-IUS should not be used as a postcoital
intrauterine contraceptive* (failures have been reported); acting
by a hormone, it appears not to act as quickly as the intrauterine copper ion does.

The relative contraindications for copper IUDs also apply to the
LNG-IUS, but are usually less strong; indeed bleeding and pain are
positive indications (WHO 1).

Duration of use of the LNG-IUS in the older woman

The product is licensed for 5 years. However, the following
should be noted:

- For *contraception*, effective use is evidence-based but
unlicensed for up to 7 years. For a woman under age 35,
because of her greater fertility, replacement after the usual 5
years would be advisable. But the *older* woman whose LNG-IUS
was fitted above the age of 35 might continue for 7 years, at
her fully empowered request (but always on a 'named-patient'
basis – p. 150). Furthermore, NICE has stated that a woman
who had her LNG-IUS inserted above the age of 45 and who
has complete amenorrhoea may continue to use the same LNG-
IUS 'until contraception is no longer needed'.
- As *part of HRT*, current practice for safe endometrial protection
would be always to change at 4 years.
- But if the LNG-IUS is *not being and will not be used for either
contraception or HRT*, it could be left in situ for as long as it
continues to work, in the control of heavy and/or painful uterine
bleeding, and then removed after ovarian failure can be finally
assured.

Conclusions – the LNG-IUS

This method fulfils many of the standard criteria for an ideal
contraceptive (see the box on pp. 6–7). It approaches 100%

reversibility, effectiveness and even, after some delay, convenience. This is because, after the initial months of frequent uterine bleedings and spotting, the usual outcomes of either intermittent light menses or amenorrhoea are very acceptable to most women. Adverse side effects are few and, in general, they are in the 'nuisance' category rather than hazardous.

However, this method does fail on some criteria: above all that it is not sufficiently protective against STIs, especially the sexually transmitted viruses, so wherever STI transmission risk applies condoms must be used in addition. We also eagerly await an implantable version, based on the GyneFix concept.

CONTRAINDICATIONS TO INTRAUTERINE CONTRACEPTION

Note that these apply to the LNG-IUS as well as to copper IUDs, except where stated.

Absolute – but perhaps temporary – contraindications (WHO 4) to fitting IUDs/LNG-IUS

- Suspicion of *pregnancy*
- Undiagnosed *irregular genital tract bleeding*
- *Significant infection*: post-septic abortion, current pelvic infection or STI, undiagnosed pelvic tenderness/deep dyspareunia or purulent cervical discharge
- *Significant immunosuppression*
- Malignant or benign *trophoblastic disease, while hCG is abnormal* (WHO 4 for IUDs and the IUS, according to UKMEC). All are agreed this becomes WHO 1 when hCG is undetectable
- (LNG-IUS *only*) *Breast cancer*, becoming WHO 3 in remission (see pp. 116–7). However, this might be an *indication* for a copper IUD
- The woman's own ethics forbidding her to use a method with a possible post-fertilization medianism (p. 127).

Absolute permanent contraindications (WHO 4) to fitting IUDs/LNG-IUS

- Markedly *distorted uterine cavity*, or cavity sounding to *less than 5.5 cm* depth (but this is only WHO 2 for GyneFix)

- Known true *allergy to a constituent*
- *Wilson's disease* (copper IUDs only)
- *Pulmonary hypertension*, because of a risk of fatal vasovagal reaction through cervical instrumentation
- Previous *endocarditis*, or after *prosthetic valve replacement* (LNG-IUS can be WHO 3 for these, as it is believed the progestogen effect on mucus reduces risk of infection leading to endocarditis – however, full anti-endocarditis antibiotic cover is required for the insertion (see point 8 in the next box).

Relative contraindications to intrauterine contraceptives – WHO 2 unless otherwise stated

This is a longish list, but in all cases meaning an IUD or the LNG-IUS is certainly usable, with some degree of caution Note again the differences specific to the LNG-IUS.

1. *Nulliparity and young age*, especially less than 20 years. Although this is WHO 2 for fear of infection and the more serious implications should that happen (with no babies yet), this just means 'broadly usable'. Both IUDs and IUSs are used successfully by many (carefully selected) women.
2. Lifestyle of self or partner(s) *risking STIs*. Combined with (1), this equates to WHO 4, rarely 3 (but only with committed condom use).
3. Past *history of definite pelvic infection*.
4. Recent *exposure to high risk of a STI* (e.g. after rape – WHO 3). In emergency situations, such as for postcoital contraception, a copper IUD may be permissible (WHO 3) with full antibiotic cover (and after microbiological swabs are taken).
5. Known *HIV infection*. While controlled by drug therapy, this is only WHO 2. LNG-IUS is better still because of reduced blood loss (added condom use is routinely advised anyway).
6. *Past history of ectopic pregnancy* or other history suggesting high ectopic risk in a *nullipara* is WHO 3, in my view, but WHO 1 (as UKMEC) if there are living children. If used, banded IUDs (eg T-Safe Cu 380A) or the IUS are best (WHO 2); but it is preferable to use an anovulant method.
7. *Suspected subfertility* already. This is WHO 2 for any cause, or WHO 3 if it relates to a tubal cause.
8. *Structural heart disease with risk of endocarditis*, but no history thereof (see above). This is WHO 3, signifying a need for full antibiotic cover for IUD or IUS insertion as advised in the BNF. LNG-IUS is probably better for these cases than a copper IUD, as it is believed to pose less ongoing infection risk due to the mucus effect.

9. *Any prosthesis* that can be prejudiced by bloodborne infection (e.g. hip replacement). IUDs are certainly usable, but are termed WHO 2 to flag up a preference for antibiotic cover for the insertion.
10. *Postpartum,* between 48 hours and 4 weeks (excess risk of perforation; WHO 3).
11. *Fibroids or congenital abnormality of the uterus* with some but not marked distortion of the uterine cavity (see above). This is WHO 2 for framed IUDs or IUSs, WHO 1 for GyneFix.
12. Severely *scarred/distorted uterus*, e.g. after myomectomy (WHO 3).
13. After *endometrial ablation/resection* – there is a risk of the IUD becoming stuck in the shrunken and scarred cavity. LNG-IUS or GyneFix are usable in selected cases.
14. *Heavy periods*, with or without anaemia before insertion for any reason, including anticoagulation. This is an indication for the LNG-IUS (WHO 1).
15. *Dysmenorrhoea, any type*. The LNG-IUS may well benefit this, provided the frame does not cause spasmodic pain.
16. *Endometriosis*. This may be benefited by the LNG-IUS (WHO 1), to help local symptoms in addition to systemic treatment.
17. *Diabetes*. This is WHO 2 for infection risk, but the IUD and LNG-IUS can be excellent choices.
18. *Penicillamine* treatment. 'Small print'; there is an unproven risk of causing copper IUD failure; the LNG-IUS not affected.
19. *Previous perforation* of uterus. This is WHO 2, almost WHO 1, at least for the small defect in the uterine fundus after a previous IUD perforation. Healing is so complete that it is usually difficult even to locate the site of the previous event.
20. (LNG-IUS only) *Liver tumour or cancer* (WHO 3 because of the systemic progestogen).

Notes
- If it is available and a copper IUD is desired, GyneFix, being frameless, would often be preferable for (11)–(13).
- The LNG-IUS is often best for (5), (8) and (13)–(18).

COUNSELLING, INSERTION AND FOLLOW-UP

Timing of insertions – all intrauterine contraceptives

Generally:

- *In the normal cycle*, timing must be planned to avoid an already implanted pregnancy, but otherwise it is a myth that insertion is best during menses (higher expulsion rates are reported then, in fact).
- *With copper IUDs* (because they are such efficient postcoital methods) insertion can be at any time up to 5 days after the calculated day of ovulation, or even:
- *At any* time in the cycle – if the provider is reasonably certain of the woman not being, nor just about to be, pregnant in a conception cycle (see p. 144).
- For the LNG-IUS, a more cautious timing policy is advised (see below).
- *Postpartum insertions* of IUD or IUSs are usually at 6 weeks and acceptable from 4 weeks (beware the increased risk of perforation). If the woman is not fully breastfeeding, conception risk should be discussed (p. 145) – and with the IUS, additional contraception is advised for 7 days.
- *Following first-trimester abortion* (but only after preliminary counselling and full agreement by the woman), immediate insertion is best:
  – On the day of surgical-induced abortion or the second part of a medical abortion, if the uterus is clearly empty – this can be checked by on-the-spot ultrasound.

Additional points about insertion timing for the LNG-IUS

- *In the normal cycle*. Insertion for the IUS should be no later than day 7 of the normal cycle, since it does not operate as an effective postcoital contraceptive *and* because, in addition, any fetus *might* be harmed by conception in the first cycle (given the *very* high local LNG concentration). *Later insertion* is also acceptable, but only if there has been believable abstinence beforehand and with continued contraception (e.g. condoms) post insertion, for 7 days.
- *If a woman is on COC or POP/Cerazette or DMPA,* the IUS can normally be inserted any time, with no added precautions.

Clinical implications

As for Implanon, insertions only in the above tiny natural-cycle window are a logistic and conception risk nightmare! So a useful practical tip is actively to recommend use of an anovulant method (i.e. one of those in the second point in the last box) at counselling, for use from then until LNG-IUS insertion. Insertion can then be at any convenient time, without any timing problems or conception anxiety.

> • Practical tip: if the COC is chosen, it may usefully be run on ('tricycled'), so that the implant is placed during already-established amenorrhoea.

Counselling and follow-up

After considering the contraindications, there should be an unhurried discussion with the woman of all the main practical points about this method, focusing on infection risk and the importance of reporting pain as a symptom at any time – and of telephoning if it occurred in the first 3 weeks post insertion.

The pre-insertion examination should usually include a *Chlamydia* screen (p. 109), and she should always be given a user-friendly back-up leaflet. She should be assured that during the use of the method, in the event of relevant symptoms or if she can no longer feel her threads, she will always receive prompt advice ('open house') and, as indicated, a pelvic examination.

The only important routine follow-up visit is at about 6 weeks after insertion. This is to:

- discuss with the woman any menstrual (or other) symptoms
- check for (partial) expulsion
- exclude infection, i.e. no relevant symptoms, tenderness or mass.

According to the WHO (and I agree), there need be no planned visits thereafter, especially no annual visits – but always with the above open-house policy.

Training for the actual insertion process

A book such as this is *not* the right medium for teaching insertion techniques. The Faculty of FP training leading to the Letter of Competence in Intrauterine Contraception Techniques is strongly recommended. This is a one-to-one apprenticeship, supplemented by videos and preliminary practice with an appropriate pelvic model, following the illustrations for each product that are in the packet.

Good analgesia is crucial – more practical tips
- Pre-medication with a prostaglandin inhibitor (e.g. mefenamic acid 500 mg or ibuprofen 400 mg) while in the waiting room, should be routine for all insertions.
- Local anaesthesia by intracervical injection should be taught and offered as a choice. It should almost always be used if the cervix has to be dilated or the uterine cavity explored.
- Moreover, there is a very unpredictable but sometimes bad pain that any woman (even a relaxed parous woman) may experience, caused by the application of the tenaculum at 12 o'clock on the cervix; and an initial 1 ml dose of 1% lidocaine completely abolishes this. So it is my practice to *offer* this to all-comers.

As we have already noted, it is worth getting all aspects of insertion training right, given the truth of: **IUD Slogan 1** (p. 101) – *Insertion can be a factor in the causation of almost every category of IUD problems*. The trainee's expertise must also be maintained thereafter, long term, through regular practice.

Postcoital contraception

Apart from mifepristone (RU486) – a 'hot potato' politically, so still unavailable for this use – three methods have now been shown to be effective contraceptives when initiated *after* unprotected sexual intercourse (UPSI):

- the insertion of a copper IUD
- the **combined oral emergency contraceptive (COEC)** using LNG 500 μg + EE 100 μg repeated in 12 hours
- the **levonorgestrel progestogen-only emergency contraceptive (LNG EC)**, given as a stat dose of LNG 1500 μg.

Marketed in the UK as Levonelle 1500, both on prescription and over-the-counter in pharmacies, LNG EC has now superseded COEC in the UK.

An important finding for both hormone methods is that delay in treatment increases the failure rate. This essentially means treating as soon as possible. But emergency contraception (EC) remains a better lay term than 'morning-after pill', since it leaves open the following facts:

- Useful benefit can be obtained long after the 'morning after' – indeed it is licensed for use post-coitally up to 72 hours and is usable even later in selected cases.
- There is a **copper IUD alternative**, which is not a 'pill' at all. See Table 10.

Importantly, there is no upper age limit to any of the methods if a sufficient risk of conception is present.

Table 10
Emergency contraception: choice of methods[a]

	LNG EC LNG 1.5 mg as stat dose	Copper IUD Immediate insertion, but sometimes better to delay (see text)
Normal timing after intercourse	Up to 72 hours but also usable up to 120 hours (see text)	Up to 5 days, or 5 days after earliest calculated day of ovulation
Efficacy (overall) within 72 hours	About 99%	About 99.9%
Side effects	Nausea 23% (15%)[b] Vomiting 6% (1.4%)[b]	Pain, bleeding, risk of infection
Contraindications (WHO 4)	• Pregnancy • Proven *severe* acute allergy to a constituent • Active acute porphyria with past attack triggered by sex hormones • Woman's own ethics precluding a possible post-fertilization mechanism	• Pregnancy • As for copper IUD generally (including *either* final point if it applies, below left)

[a]WHO. *Lancet* 1998; **352**: 428–4.).
[b]WHO. *Lancet* 2002; **360**: 1803–10 (this study showed a lower rate of side effects in the parentheses).

Levonorgestrel emergency contraception (LNG EC)

Mechanism of action

Given at or before ovulation, *the method:*

* interferes with follicle development, either inhibiting altogether or possibly *delaying* ovulation – *clinically*, impress therefore on any user the continuing conception risk from unprotected sex post-treatment
* rapidly makes the cervical mucus hostile to sperm.

Given later in a cycle, it is:

* believed to be also capable of inhibiting implantation, but this seems to be the less effective of its mechanisms – so the failure rate tends to be higher for sexual exposures late in the cycle.

Effectiveness and advantages of LNG EC

The 1998 randomised controlled trial (RCT) by WHO has now been amplified by a larger RCT totalling 4136 women in 10 countries. In the latter there was randomization to mifepristone and either to LNG 1500 μg stat or to the same total dose in divided doses of 750 μg taken 12 hours apart [WHO (2002) von Hertzen et al. *Lancet* 2002; **360**: 1803–10]. No difference in efficacy nor in side-effects was detectable between the two LNG regimens.

Main advantages of LNG EC:
- Greater effectiveness: 99.6% when treatment began *within 24 hours of a single exposure*, compared with 98% for COEC – in the circumstances of the 1998 WHO trial
- Reduced rates of the main side effects of nausea and vomiting
- In ordinary practice, virtually no contraindications.

The apparent effectiveness of LNG EC with treatment up to 72 hours after a single sexual exposure is around 99% – but this represents prevention of only 80% of the expected pregnancies, since most of those who present would not actually have conceived. Moreover, in the real world, multiple acts of UPSI without 'perfect' condom use both before and after the treatment can greatly increase the conception risk.

Enzyme-inducer drug (EID) treatment

If the woman is taking one of these (listed on p. 50; also bosentan, p. 71), hormonal EC is WHO 3. As usual, this category means that it would be better to use an alternative, in this case:

- insertion of a copper IUD (the most effective option), or
- if that is not acceptable, the dose should be doubled i.e. two tablets totalling 3 mg stat (unlicensed use – p. 150).

The same applies if the woman is currently taking St John's Wort ('Nature's Prozac'), which is an enzyme-inducer. But no increase in dose is needed when non-enzyme-inducing antibiotics are in use.

Warfarin-users should have their INR checked in 3–4 days after LNG EC, since it may alter significantly.

Contraindications to LNG EC

Absolute contraindications (WHO 4) to the hormone methods are essentially non-existent (WHOMEC) – in my view (differing slightly from UKMEC), those that might be so classified are:

- Current pregnancy (as it would be pointless anyway: *but*, if LNG EC were given in error, it is not thought that the pregnancy would be harmed at all)
- Proven severe allergy or intolerance to a constituent
- Active acute porphyria, if a past attack was precipitated by sex hormones
- If the woman's own ethics, on discussion, preclude intervention post-coitally (or more relevantly, post-fertilization) – i.e. she disagrees with the UK legal view (see below).

Relative contraindications
- EID treatment, see above (WHO 3) – copper IUD better
- Current breast cancer (WHO 2 due to uncertainty, but an adverse effect is unlikely with such short exposure) and
- Trophoblastic disease with high hCG levels (WHO 2)
- Current active and severe liver disease (WHO 3).

Breastfeeding is not a contraindication, although the conception risk is of course usually (p. 70) so low that EC treatment would rarely be needed. If it is indicated, the infant should not be harmed in any way by the tiny amount of LNG reaching the breast milk, especially if, as a 2006 study showed, there are no feeds from the breast for just 8 hours after the EC dose.

Copper intrauterine devices

Insertion of a copper IUD – *not* the LNG IUS (see p. 117) – before implantation is extremely effective, through the toxicity of copper ions to sperm or by blocking implantation. This means, after consultation with the woman, that insertion may proceed *in good faith*, up to 5 days after:

- the first sexual exposure (regardless of cycle length); **or**
- the (earliest) calculated ovulation day – this requires one to:
  - calculate the *soonest likely* next menstrual start day
  - subtract 14 days for mean life of the corpus luteum
  - add 5 days to allow for the mean interval from fertilization to implantation.

The judge's summing up in a 1991 Court Case (*Regina* vs *Dhingra*) gives legal support to thus intervening up to 5 days post-ovulation/fertilization:

> '*I further hold ... that a pregnancy cannot come into existence until the fertilized ovum has become implanted in the womb, and that that stage is not reached until, at the earliest, the 20th day of a normal 28 day cycle...*'

Similarly, the conclusion of the Judicial Review of Emergency Contraception in 2002 confirmed the long-held position of most ethicists who considered the matter – namely that a pregnancy begins at implantation, not when an egg is fertilized.

Effectiveness of copper IUD

The copper IUD prevents conception in well over 99% of women who present, or 98% of those who might be expected otherwise to conceive: even in cases of multiple exposure ever since the last menstrual period.

Indications for EC by copper IUD

In selected individuals, IUD insertion may be preferable to oral EC:

- When maximum efficacy is the woman's priority – her choice. UKMEC says it should be *offered* to all – even to those presenting within 72 hours.
- When exposure occurred more than 72 hours earlier, or in cases of multiple exposure: insertion may be:
  - up to 5 days after the earliest UPSI, or
  - if there have been many UPSI acts, no later than 5 days after ovulation.
- In many women – often, though not always, parous – when it is to be retained as their long-term method (although it may be appropriate in many young women to remove it after their next menses, once they are established on a new method such as the COC or injectable). Always try to insert a banded IUD where long-term use is a possibility.
- In the presence of contraindications to the hormonal method (very rare with LNG EC, but enzyme-inducer drugs are WHO 3 – so consider an IUD).
- If the woman is currently in a vomiting attack when she presents, *or* unexpectedly vomits her dose of LNG EC within 2 hours in a case with particularly high pregnancy risk.

Contraindications to the IUD method and clinical implications

The IUD method has a number of recognized contraindications (pp 116–20) and always risks pain, bleeding or post-insertion infection. So this option should be reserved for those with one of the above special indications.

Clinically, given the likely sexual history (p. 6), when taken, insertion in most cases should be:

- after microbiological cervical screening (at least for *Chlamydia trachomatis*)
- with prophylactic antibiotic cover, e.g. with azithromycin 1 g stat
- with contact tracing to follow if STI test results later prove positive.

Insertion might be expected to be difficult in a nullipara, but rarely needs to be off the day of presentation. It can usually be arranged later after referral to a skilled clinician at a nearby Level 2 service, given the ability to use IUDs late in the cycle, up to 5 days after ovulation (see above), on day 17, but for a woman with a 26-day shortest cycle, inserting say on day 14 after high-risk UPSI on day 11.

In such cases, UKMEC recommends giving LNG EC on the day of presentation, as a holding manoeuvre.

Summary: counselling and management of EC cases

First, evaluate the possibility of sexual abuse or rape. Then, **in a context that preserves confidentiality** – and feels that way to the client – using (crucially) a good leaflet, such as that of the FPA, as the basis for discussion, help the woman to make a fully informed and autonomous choice. This could be *either* of the two EC methods, *or*, in some rare circumstances, taking no post coital action at all.

Pharmacists should ensure privacy for the discussion and have a low threshold to refer all cases outside their specified remit (e.g. more than 72 hours since the earliest UPSI) to an appropriate clinical provider.

Clinical management

- Careful assessment of *menstrual/coital history* is essential. Probe for other exposures to risk earlier than the one presented with. Note: ovulation is such a variable event and LNG EC is so safe that most women are best treated whenever they present – in the 'normal' cycle. Note that this is in marked contrast to the Pill cycle (below).
- *Assess contraindications*. The mode of action may itself pose the only contraindication/problem, for some individuals. Sometimes, it may help to explain that there are circumstances when the powerful pre-fertilization effects of LNG EC can remove concern about it needing to use the post-fertilization mechanism (e.g. if the treatment is clearly going to be given well before ovulation in a given cycle – despite being post-coitus).
- *Medical risks* may be a concern, and should be set out in the information leaflet that is given, especially:
  - The *failure rate* (see above): remind the woman that the WHO figures relate to a single exposure. The failure rate is close to nil for the IUD method.
  - *Teratogenicity:* this is believed to be negligible – although there is no proof – because before implantation the hormones will not reach the blastocyst in sufficient concentration to cause any adverse effect. Follow-up of women who have kept their pregnancies has so far not shown any increased risk of major abnormalities above the background rate of 2%.
  - *Ectopic pregnancy:* if this occurs, as it may, the EC was not causative. It results from a pre-existing damaged tube and would almost certainly have happened anyway, with or without this (pre-implantation) treatment. However:

    a past history of ectopic pregnancy or pelvic infection remains a reason for specific forewarning with any EC method

    all women should be warned to report back urgently if they get **pain** – and providers must 'think ectopic' whenever LNG EC or a copper IUD fails, or there is an unusual bleeding pattern post-treatment.
- *Side-effects:* in the WHO 2002 trial, nausea occurred in 15% and vomiting in 1.4% of users. If the contraceptive dose is vomited within 2 hours, instead of an IUD the woman may be given a further tablet with an anti-emetic: the best seems to be domperidone (Motilium) 10 mg.
- *Contraception,* both in the current cycle (in case the LNG EC

method merely postpones ovulation) – often condoms – and in the long term, should be discussed. The IUD option may cover both aspects (for a suitable long-term user). Inform the woman that by the end of a year, regular use of almost any approved method will give better efficacy than using EC every month. If the COC or injectable is chosen, it should normally be started as soon as the woman is convinced her next period is normal – usually on the first or second day – without the need for additional contraception thereafter.

- But *'Quick start' of the COC is also an option* in selected cases. This means starting a COC immediately after the EC along with advice for 7 days of added condom use and hopefully 100% follow-up. The clinician must be confident that the benefits (especially the greater probability of future compliance) outweigh the risks of EC failure. 'Quick start' is unlicensed, so should be on a 'named-patient' basis (p. 150), with appropriate documented warnings.

The above description highlights the importance of a good rapport, to obtain an honest and accurate coital/menstrual history and to promote arrangements for more effective contraception in future.

Follow-up

Women receiving LNG EC (except with 'Quick start') are rarely seen again routinely, but should be instructed to return:

- if they experience pain, or
- their expected period is more than 7 days late, or lighter than usual.

IUD-acceptors return usually in 4–6 weeks for a routine check-up; or perhaps for device removal, once established on what for them is a more appropriate long-term method.

Special indications for EC

These apply to coital exposure when the following have occurred:
- **Omission of anything more than two COC tablets after the PFI, or of more than two pills in the first seven in the packet** (see p. 45). As explained there, after the first pill-taking week,

since seven tablets have been taken to render the ovules quiescent, pill-omissions almost never indicate emergency treatment. Moreover, towards the end of a packet (pill-days 15–21), simple omission of the next PFI will always suffice (no matter how many pills have been missed, up to the seven in that week!).

- **Delay in taking a POP tablet for more than 3 hours**, outside of lactation, implying loss of the mucus effect, or of a Cerazette tablet for more than 12 hours, followed by sexual exposure before mucus-based contraception was restored (in 2 days – p. 70). The POP or Cerazette is restarted immediately after the emergency regimen, 2 days' added precautions are advised, and follow-up agreed.

- **If the POP-user is breastfeeding,** emergency contraception would only be indicated if either the breastfeeding or the POP-taking were unusually inadequate (p. 70)!

- **Removal or expulsion of an IUD** before the time of implantation, if another IUD cannot be inserted, for some reason.

- **Further exposure in the same natural cycle** – e.g. due to failure of barrier contraception more than 1 day after a dose of EC has been taken. Additional courses of LNG EC are supported by UKMEC, 'if clinically indicated', given reasonable precautions to avoid treating after implantation (yet repeated use thereafter will not induce an abortion). This use is, again, outside the terms of the licence (see p. 150).

- **Use of LNG EC later than 72 hours after earliest UPSI.** In a randomized controlled trial by the WHO (2002), the failure rate was low, with only 8 failures in 314 women treated between 72 and 120 hours (5 days) after the earliest act of unprotected intercourse. WHO concluded this is 'prevention of a high proportion of pregnancies even up to 5 days after coitus'. But the confidence intervals were wide, also other data suggest the prime mechanism that hormonal EC uses is to stop or delay ovulation and it probably rarely operates by implantation-block after fertilization. Therefore, if the risk may have been taken during the approx 5 days between fertilization and implantation, it is usually unwise to use the LNG method of EC later than 72 hours after intercourse. With that *timing* caveat, use up to 5 days post coitus is acceptable as an example of **evidence-based but *unlicensed* use of a licensed product (see p. 150)**. Women should be told of the limited evidence of efficacy – 'likely to be better than doing nothing' – and also informed that a copper IUD would definitely be more effective (and is usable up to 5 days after the calculated ovulation day (pp. 127–8) *regardless of the number of unprotected sexual acts up to that time*).

- **Overdue injections of DMPA with continuing sexual intercourse** (see p. 82). If it is later than day 91 (end of the 13th week) then LNG EC may be given along with the next injection **plus** advice to use condoms for 7 days. But after day 98 (14 weeks), the next injection is best postponed until there has been a total of 14 days of safe contraception or abstinence since the last exposure and a sensitive (<25 mIU/l) pregnancy test is negative – again with 7 days' added precautions and good follow-up.
- **Advanced provision of LNG EC**: UKMEC supports this in selected cases, to increase early use when required – e.g. to cover the risk of condom rupture or refusal of the partner to use when travelling abroad.

In all circumstances of use of EC, the women should be aware (as stated in the FPA leaflet) that

- The method might fail
- It is not an abortifacient
- It is given too soon to be able to harm a baby.

Research continues, and new alternatives may supersede the current methods in due course.

Other reversible methods *

BARRIER METHODS

Barrier methods are not yet out of fashion! In spite of well-known disadvantages, they all (notably condoms) provide useful protection against STIs. *All users of this type of method should be informed about EC, in case of lack of use or failure in use.*

Vegetable- and oil-based lubricants, and the bases for many prescribable vaginal products, can seriously damage and lead to rupture of rubber: baby oil destroys up to 95% of a condom's strength within 15 minutes. Beware ad hoc use of, or contamination by, substances from the kitchen or bathroom cupboard! Water-based products such as KY Jelly, and also glycerine and silicone lubricants, are not suspect. The box on p. 135 lists some common vaginal preparations that should be regarded as unsafe to use with rubber condoms and diaphragms – and there may be others.

This problem does not affect plastic condoms such as Avanti and Ez-On (see below). However, there is no evidence that either of these is any less likely to rupture for mechanical reasons.

---

*Male and female sterilization – especially the former, which is more effective – are useful options for some couples, but are not within the remit of this particular book.

Condoms

Condoms are the only proven barrier to transmission of HIV – yet, at the time of writing, it still remains impossible in the UK for most couples to obtain this life-saver free of charge from every GP. Condoms are second in usage to the Pill among those under the age of 30 and to sterilization above that age. One GP has reported a failure rate as low as 0.4 per 100 woman-years, but 2–15 is more representative. Failure, often unrecognized at the time, can almost always be attributed to incorrect use – mainly through escape of a small amount of semen either before or after the main ejaculation. Conceptions – particularly among the young or those who have become a bit casual after years of using a simple method such as the COC – can sometimes be iatrogenic because of lack of explanation by a nurse or doctor of the basics.

Some users are entirely satisfied with the condom, whereas others use it as a temporary or back-up method. For many who have become accustomed to alternatives not related to intercourse, it is completely unacceptable. Some older men, or those with sexual anxiety, complain that its use may result in loss of erection. I consider this sometimes gives adequate grounds to prescribe sildenafil. For women who dislike the smell or messiness of semen, the condom solves their problem.

True rubber allergy can also occur (rarely), but is often solved by switching to plastic condoms (e.g. Avanti or Ez-On). If the allergy proves to be to the lubricant, if it contains nonoxinol-9, it should not be being used in the first place. Lubricants with this spermicide should be avoided with any condom, since there is now evidence that it can increase HIV transmission (see below) – and, anyway, it provides no detectable increase in condom efficacy.

The Ez-On condom and its variants

Available in California and the Netherlands (and hopefully soon in the UK), this is a loose-fitting well-lubricated plastic condom – the 'looks funny, feels good' condom. In some respects, it is the concept of the female condom 'put back on the man'. By a better simulation of the normal vagina, it is designed to overcome the undeniable interference with penile sensation that occurs during the penetrative phase of intercourse.

Femidom

Femidom (Figure 17) is a female condom comprising a polyurethane sac with an outer rim at the introitus and a loose inner ring, whose retaining action is similar to that of the rim of the diaphragm. It thus forms a well-lubricated secondary vagina. Available over the counter, along with a well-illustrated leaflet, it is completely resistant to damage by any chemicals with which it

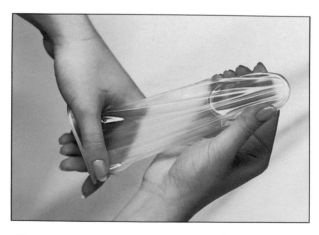

Figure 17
The female condom (Femidom). (Reproduced with kind permission of Chartex International plc.)

might come into contact. Using it, the penetrative phase of inter-course can feel more normal (as with Ez-On) and also start before the man's erection is complete. However, couples should be forewarned of the possibility that the penis may become wrongly positioned between the Femidom sac and the vaginal wall.

Reports about its acceptability are mixed, and a sense of humour certainly helps. There is evidence of a group of women (and their partners) who use it regularly, sometimes alternating with the male equivalent ('his' night then 'her' night). Others might choose it if it were more often mentioned by providers as even being an option. As the first female-controlled method with high potential for preventing HIV transmission, it must be welcomed.

The cap or diaphragm

Once initiated, many couples express surprise at the simplicity of these vaginal barriers, although they are often acceptable only when sexual activity takes on a relatively regular pattern in a stable relationship (and nowadays usually above age 35). The cap may be inserted well ahead of coitus, and so used without spoiling spontaneity. There is very little reduction in sexual sensitivity, as the clitoris and introitus are not affected and cervi-cal pressure is still possible.

Spermicide is recommended because no mechanical barrier is complete, although we still lack definitive research on this point. Possible toxic effects of nonoxinol-9 – which is unfortunately the only spermicidal agent marketed in UK – to the vaginal wall have become a real concern (see below). However, the vagina is believed to be able to recover between applications when nonoxinol-9 is used in the manner, and at the kind of average coital frequency, of typical diaphragm-users.

The acceptability of the *diaphragm* itself depends on how it is offered. Its first-year failure rate, now estimated as high as 4–8 per 100 careful and consistent users, rising to 10–18 per 100 typical users, makes it very unsuitable for most young women who would not accept pregnancy. However, it suits others who are 'spacers' of their family. And it is capable of excellent protection above the age of 35 (3 per 100 woman-years, as the Oxford/FPA study reported in the early 1980s), provided it is as well taught and correctly and consistently used as it was by those couples.

Lea's Shield and *Femcap* are both American inventions. The latter has some efficacy data; the reported Pearl failure rate is comparable with that of the diaphragm: 10.5–14.5 per 100 woman-years. It is a plastic cervical cap with a brim filling the fornices, in three sizes, intended to be provided through mainstream clinics (supplier: Durbin) as an alternative to the diaphragm or cervical caps. It must be used with a spermicide, but is reusable, needing to be replaced about every 2 years.

When there is great difficulty in inserting anything into the vagina – be it tampon, pessaries or a cap – the method is obviously not suitable. This problem may be connected with a psycho-sexual difficulty that may first present during the teaching of the method, but simple lack of anatomical knowledge is often involved. Rejection of a vaginal barrier on account of 'messi-ness' may also be the result of such a problem.

Follow-up

Vaginal barriers should be checked initially after 1–2 weeks of trial, then annually. The fitting of diaphragms should be re-checked routinely postpartum, or if there is a 4 kg gain or loss in weight.

If either partner returns complaining that they can feel any kind of cap during coitus, the fitting must be urgently checked. It could be too large or too small; or with the diaphragm the retro-pubic ledge may be insufficient to prevent the front slipping down the anterior vagina; or, most seriously, the item may be being placed regularly in the anterior fornix. The *arcing spring diaphragm* is then particularly useful.

Chronic cystitis may be exacerbated by pressure from a diaphragm's anterior rim, and the condition was shown to occur less frequently with *Femcap* in the comparative pre-marketing trials. Similarly, it often improves with a *vault* or *cervical cap*.

As for the IUD, for those nurses or doctors who wish to offer this choice, there is no substitute for one-to-one training, both in the process of fitting the diaphragm and cervical caps and in teaching a woman how to use it correctly, backed by an appropriate leaflet

With each of these products, the single most important thing the woman must learn is the vital regular secondary check, after placing it, that she has covered her cervix correctly. Female barriers can be used happily and very successfully by many couples, but high motivation is essential. Once again, a good sense of humour helps.

Spermicides

Sadly, many useful products such as Delfen foam and Gynol II jelly have now been removed from the UK market. At the time of writing, the only products available are Orthoform pessaries and Ortho Creme™ for use with diaphragms. However, the contraceptive sponge is apparently due back on the market in 2007 as the Today sponge - for details visit www.todayswomencare.com). It has the advantages of being sexually very convenient and unobtrusive in use.

Although invaluable as adjuncts to caps and diaphragms, used alone spermicides are usually not acceptably reliable. Yet spermicides and sponges can be used successfully by women whose natural fertility is reduced, particularly with increasing age,

---

The Today sponge, or other spermicidal products may be good choices in the following cases:

- For women over 50 years of age if still experiencing bleeds after stopping the COC (see pp. 147); and for 1 year after the menopause (when contraception is still advised), whether or not they use HRT
- For women aged over 45 if they have oligo-amenorrhoea
- During lactation as an alternative to the POP
- During continuing secondary amenorrhoea, unless a COC is being used anyway to treat hypoestrogenism
- As an adjunct to other contraception – e.g. spermicides may be useful as a supplement in couples who choose to continue using withdrawal as their main method
- For 'spacers', nearly but not quite ready for a first or subsequent child.

Many substances are well absorbed from the vagina, but there is no proof of systemic harm, congenital malformations or spontaneous abortions from the use of current spermicides, chiefly nonoxinol-9 or its close relatives.

Occasionally, sensitivity to a spermicide arises. More seriously, when used by Nairobi prostitutes four times a day for 14 days, nonoxinol-9 released from pessaries caused erythema and colposcopic evidence of minor damage to the vaginal skin. Coupled with the doubts about its effectiveness against intra-cellular virus, it clearly should not be promoted as an anti-HIV virucide (see the systematic review by D Wilkinson et al *Lancet Inf Dis* 2002; **2**: 613–17). However, pending better alternatives, for the time being it remains good practice to continue to recom-mend nonoxinol-9 for *normal contraceptive use* (less frequently than four times a day!), whether alone or with diaphragms or cervical caps; but *not* with condoms.

Final comment

Worldwide, there remains a great unmet need for an effective user-friendly female-controlled vaginal microbicide, which might or might not also be a spermicide. Many international agencies are now actively involved, but progress is slow in this urgent and previously neglected area of research.

FERTILITY AWARENESS AND METHODS FOR NATURAL REGULATION OF FERTILITY

At one time, these methods were generally despised and only adopted by those with strong religious views. Modern multiple index versions (based primarily on carefully charting changes to cervical mucus, the cervix itself by auto-palpation, and body temperature, with support from the so-called secondary indica-tors such as ovulation pain) are increasingly demanded by those who prefer to use a more 'natural' method. There is no space here to do justice to this approach, but there is a website that is uniquely good among all those in the area: www.fertilityuk.org. It is completely neutral. Indeed, it makes the following excellent comment regarding other information sources: '*NFP* [natural family planning] *instruction often comes with a religious orienta-tion that you may or may not appreciate*'.

Those who wish to use these methods deserve careful explanation and ideally one-to-one teaching, particularly about charting the clinical changes and the possible added use of other minor clinical indicators of fertility. Useful instruction leaflets, further advice and details of NFP teachers (mostly non-NHS) available in different locations, can be obtained from www.fertilityuk.org (and also from the FPA website, www.fpa.org.uk). Additionally they give advice about fertility awareness to assist conception.

With 'perfect use', the multiple index methods are indeed capable of being acceptably effective. However in the words of Professor Trussell of Princeton, they still remain 'very unforgiving of imperfect use'. Moreover, imperfect use is unfortunately common in the real world. To be effective, many days of abstinence are inevitable and the highest possible cooperation from both parties is required but often lacking -- especially from the male, whose motivation may well be suspect. (In one study, the failure rate was noted to be higher when the man rather than his partner was the one in charge of interpreting the temperature charts!) To be fair to the methods, failures also commonly result from poor use of other contraceptives, such as the condom, by those who do not wish to abstain during 'unsafe' days.

Persona (Unipath Ltd) (Figure 18) is a combination of mini-laboratory and microcomputer. Persona displays the 'safe' (green) and 'unsafe' (red) days of a woman's cycle, based on measurements of the first significant rise in her levels of urinary estrone-3-glucuronide and luteinising hormone. With a reduced number of 'unsafe' days (8–10 for most women) being signalled per cycle, this contraceptive option is found by many couples to make things easier – but it does not apparently lead to greater effectiveness than careful charting of the indices with good compliance. The data on the failure rate are reported as 6 per 100 woman-years in the first year even with 'perfect use' – and Trussell (personal communication, 2003) still considers this to be an underestimate.

Even on that slightly uncertain basis, couples should be informed that this is the same as a 1 in 17 risk of conceiving in

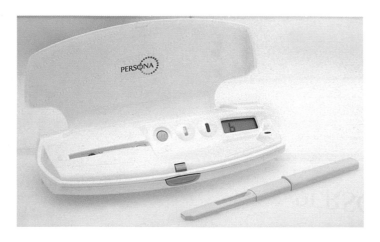

Figure 18
Persona (by courtesy of Unipath Ltd).

the first year – perhaps good enough for 'spacers'.

For greater efficacy, couples should be advised:
- to use condoms on the pre-ovulatory 'green days' – this being what I would prefer to call the 'amber' phase (always less 'safe' because of the capriciousness of sperm survival in a woman)
- to abstain completely on all 'red days'
- to have unprotected intercourse only in the post-ovulatory green phase.

Moreover, if Persona or another natural method is to be commenced after *any pregnancy* or *any hormone treatment* – even just one course of hormonal EC – reliability demands that another method such as condoms or abstinence must first be used until there have been two normal cycles of an acceptable length (23–35 days).

Lactation within the specific guidelines of the lactational amenorrhoea method (LAM) as shown in Figure 19 constitutes a quintessentially 'natural method' – through to 6 months postpartum. See also p. 70.

Ask the mother:

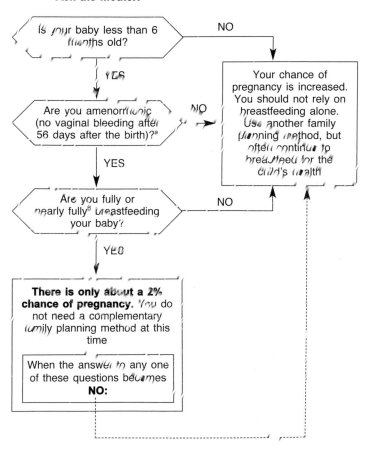

Is your baby less than 6 months old? — NO → Your chance of pregnancy is increased. You should not rely on breastfeeding alone. Use another family planning method, but often continue to breastfeed for the child's health

YES

Are you amenorrhoeic (no vaginal bleeding after 56 days after the birth)?[a] — NO →

YES

Are you fully or nearly fully[b] breastfeeding your baby? — NO →

YES

There is only about a 2% chance of pregnancy. You do not need a complementary family planning method at this time

When the answer to any one of these questions becomes **NO:**

[a]Spotting that occurs during the first 56 days is not considered to be menstruation
[b]'Nearly' full breastfeeding means that the baby obtains almost 100% of its nutrition from the mother alone, and certainly no solid food

Figure 19
Algorithm for the lactational amenorrhoea method (LAM)

Special considerations

How can a provider be reasonably sure that a woman is not pregnant, or just about to be pregnant in a conception cycle?

WHOSPR advises that the provider can be reasonably certain that the woman is not pregnant if she has no symptoms or signs of pregnancy and one or more of the following criteria apply:

1. She has not had intercourse since last normal menses
2. She has been correctly and consistently using a reliable [sic] method of contraception
3. She is within the first 7 days after (onset of) normal menses
4. She is within 4 weeks postpartum for non-lactating women
5. She is within the first 7 days post abortion or miscarriage
6. She is fully or nearly fully breastfeeding (as in LAM – Figure 19, p. 143), amenorrhoeic and less than 6 months postpartum.

Note: Good clinical judgement is vital with respect to assessing the accuracy of the given history, including:

- the absence of symptoms of pregnancy
- the believability of reported abstinence
- especially regarding point 2 in the list, reliability of reported correct condom use is notoriously difficult to assess.

In the UK, as appropriate, these criteria can be backed by a urine pregnancy test with a sensitivity of at least 25 IU/l, best on a concentrated early morning sample. Such tests are unnecessary and wasteful if there could not possibly yet be an implanted blastocyst present – including, for example, at the time of most requests for EC (e.g. in pill-takers when pills have just been missed).

Some applications of the above

Quick start

This means immediate starting of (usually) a pill method at first visit, late in the menstrual cycle or straight after EC. This may often be an entirely appropriate though unlicensed use (p. 150), but only when the above criteria have been applied, so that the provider is reasonably sure of a woman neither being nor just about to be pregnant.

Secondary amenorrhoea, wants to (re-)start contraception

This is where the greatest difficulty arises – for example:

* postpartum, not breastfeeding and beyond 4 weeks (time of first recorded ovulations) without reliable contraception to date, or
* a woman more than 2 weeks overdue with her DMPA injection.

A pair of visits may often be required, since a pre-diagnosable pregnancy (unimplanted blastocyst) might be present at the first.

First visit

Take history of early symptoms of pregnancy (increased micturition, nausea) and do a urine pregnancy test with sensitivity at least 25 IU/l (only) if the history is suggestive. If this test is negative (or there are no symptoms so it is not done) but more assurance is required before taking action as for example before inserting an LNG-IUS:

* recommend her to abstain (preferable), or
* teach her to use a back-up method such as condoms with exceptional care (greater care than ever in her life before!), or
* if neither of the above are appropriate, given that POPs have never been suspected of harming an early pregnancy, one of these may be prescribed

Until at least 14 days have elapsed since whenever was her last unprotected intercourse

She should normally return at that time, bringing an early morning urine sample. But if a pill method is planned, she may be given supplies in case her period comes on and she can start it routinely at home.

A final wise precaution

Given that in 10–15% of cases a sensitive pregnancy test 14 days post-coitally can be falsely negative, arrange for a further follow-up in 2–4 weeks to confirm her non-pregnant state. Or at least instruct the woman to return if she develops symptoms that could be pregnancy – or if she fails to see her first withdrawal bleed on the COC.

Contraception for the older woman

Duration of use of COCs

Among the *benefits* listed on pp. 13–14, most are enhanced as the duration of COC use increases. However, for *risks*, available data suggest that age seems a more important factor affecting risk than duration of use.

Maximum age for COC use

Smokers or others with arterial risk factors should always discontinue the COC at age 35 (WHO 4). Pending more data, if they request a *hormonal* contraceptive they should consider:

- a progestogen-only pill or implant, but
- an IUD or IUS would be even better; or:
- should the partner now consider having a vasectomy?

But in selected ***healthy migraine-free, non-smokers,*** with modern pills and careful monitoring, the many gynaecological and other benefits of COCs are now felt to outweigh the small, though increasing, cardiovascular and breast cancer risks (p. 14 and pp. 20–33) of a modern pill up to age 50–51, which is the mean age of the menopause. Although there are usually better contraceptive choices – consider especially an intrauterine method – an appropriate COC (usually a 20 µg product) may therefore be used till then. For women with diminishing ovarian function but who need contraception as well, this is logical and may be preferable to hormone-replacement therapy (HRT) along with having to use some other contraceptive.

But not after the 50th year, see below.

Beyond 50–51 years of age, the age-related increased COC risks are usually unacceptable for all, given that fertility is now so low that simple, virtually risk-free contraceptives will suffice – e.g. spermicides or the contraceptive sponge (p. 139)

Most forms of HRT are not contraceptive, but may be indicated combined with any such simple contraceptive in symptomatic women when estrogen is no longer being supplied by the COC. Of course, the IUS-plus-HRT combination is a winner here, since it safely supplies contraceptive HRT with endometrial protection plus, usually, also highly acceptable oligo-amenorrhoea.

The actual and expected advantages of HRT by LNG-IUS (note: change at 4 years) plus estrogen by any route
- Contraceptive HRT
- No-period, usually no-bleed HRT – before proof of ovarian failure
- No heavy/painful loss HRT, or other menstrual symptoms
- Minimal systemic progestogen HRT
  - Might be better for breast cancer risk (as progestogens can affect this), although there is no proof as yet
- Plus still giving the expected quality-of-life benefits of HRT.

Diagnosing loss of fertility at the menopause
Although hormones including the POP tend to mask the menopause, it is not always necessary to know the precise time of final ovarian failure. Moreover follicle-stimulating hormone (FSH) levels are unreliable for diagnosis of complete loss of ovarian function. So one of the options in the Box should be followed

---

Plan A *Contraception may cease: after waiting for the 'officially approved' 1 year of amenorrhoea above age 50, having stopped all hormones*

This is the obvious plan for:
- Copper IUDs
- condoms
- sponge or spermicides (which unlike in younger women appear to be adequate in the presence of such drastically reduced – progressing to absent – fertility).

But what to do if the woman is using one of the hormonal methods or HRT, which mask the menopause?

- If on DMPA or COC (or Evra patch): age 50 is the time to stop these (and maybe switch to a POP). They are needlessly strong, contraceptively, and the known risks increase with age.
- The POP, or an implant, or the LNG-IUS, or a sponge/ spermicide with ongoing HRT: as contraceptives these add negligible medical risks that increase with age – even to age 60!
- Therefore one of these (usually the POP) may be continued until the latest age of potential fertility has been reached: then the woman just stops the contraception (no tests!). When is that?
  - A good estimate is age 55. The Faculty of FP in their guidance (*J Fam Plann Reprod Health Care* 1995;**31**:51–63) quote Treloar's evidence that 95.9% have ceased menstruation for ever by then (and such bleeds as may happen later, in the other 4.1%, would be extremely unlikely to occur in cycles that were fertile).

Plan B *Contraception may cease: at age 55 after having switched to, or having continued with a progestogen-only method – most commonly a POP (old type)*

- It is true that the *Guinness Book of Records* has reported one or two older mothers (into their early 60s!), but authentication is uncertain.
- If this remains a source of anxiety there is an option, even after stopping the POP at age 55, to transfer to using a sponge or spermicide for one final year.

Plan C *Contraception may cease: above age 50 if three other criteria also apply*

Older users of hormonal contraception may cease using any method *IF:*

1. They have passed their 50th birthday, **AND**, after a trial of 2 months' discontinuation using barriers or spermicides, they have:
2. Vasomotor symptoms
3. Two separate high FSH levels (>30 U/l) when off all treatment
4. Continuing amenorrhoea thereafter

> With due warnings of lack of certainty, these women may cease all
> contraception earlier than the approved 1 year post 50. Or, as
> before, just use a sponge or spermicide for one final year.

There are useful clues for COC-users and POP-users that
discontinuation to follow the protocol in the above box is worth
a try, namely;

- if COC-users start getting 'hot flushes' at the end of their
  pill-free interval – especially if a high FSH result is
  obtained then
- if old-type POP-users develop vasomotor symptoms with
  amenorrhoea (see p. 77).

Appendix

USE OF LICENSED PRODUCTS IN AN UNLICENSED WAY

Often, licensing procedures have not yet caught up with what is widely considered the best evidence-based practice, Such use is legitimate and may indeed be necessary for optimal contraceptive care, provided certain criteria are observed. These are well established (see FFPRHC Guidance July 2005. *J Fam Plann Reprod Health Care* 2005;**31**:225–42).

The prescribing physician must accept full liability and:
- Be adopting an evidence-based practice endorsed by a responsible body of professional opinion
- *Assess the individual's priorities and preferences,* giving a clear account of known and possible risks and the benefits
- *Explain to her that it is an unlicensed prescription*
- *Obtain informed (verbal) consent and record this*
- Ensure good practice, including follow-up, to comply fully with professional indemnity requirements: along with meticulous record-keeping
- *Note that this will often mean the doctor providing dedicated written materials*, because the manufacturer's PIL insert may not apply in one or more respects.

This protocol is generally termed **'named-patient' prescribing**.

Note

1. Attention to detail is important – as in the (unlikely) event of a claim, the manufacturer can be excused from any liability.
2. *Nurse prescribers* cannot *prescribe* medicines outside the terms of the licence, but they may supply and administer

them as above, within fully agreed and authorized Patient Group Directions (and as agreed with their insurer, such as the Royal College of Nursing).

Some common examples of named-patient prescribing
- Advising more than the usual dosage, such as when enzyme-inducer drugs are being used with:
  - the COC or POP (Cerazette, p. 71) or
  - hormonal emergency contraception
- Sustained use of COC over many cycles:
  - long-term tricycling or, now:
  - 365/365 use (p. 48)
- Use of banded copper IUDs for longer than licensed:
  - under the age of 40 (e.g. T-Safe Cu 380A for more than 10 years, GyneFix for more than 5 years)
  - continuing use to post-menopause of *any* copper device that was fitted after age 40
- Continuing use of the same LNG-IUS for contraception:
  - in an older woman (e.g. where fitted above 35) for up to 7 years rather than the licensed 5 years, at a patient's fully informed request
  - indefinitely if fitted above 45 and she is amenorrhoeic (NICE advice)
- Use of hormonal EC:
  - beyond 72 hours after the earliest exposure
  - or more than once in a cycle
- *Use of 'Quick start'.* This means, with appropriate safeguards (including applying the criteria on p. 144 to reduce conception risk), commencement of pills or other medical methods of contraception:
  - late in the menstrual cycle
  - or immediately after hormonal EC.

There are other examples that may be identified elsewhere in this book, as well as in the Faculty of FP guidance referenced above.

EQUIVALENT PROPRIETARY NAMES FOR COMBINED PILLS WORLDWIDE

In previous editions of this book, the above directory appeared in printed form. It listed details of the equivalent brand names used worldwide, identical with or very similar to currently marketed UK low-dose combined pills. The International

Planned Parenthood Federation (IPPF) now has this directory in its entirety on its website. This is accessible to all (no password), accurate, and regularly updated: www.ippf.org.uk.

BELIEVABLE WEBSITES IN REPRODUCTIVE HEALTH

www.margaretpyke.org
Local services and superb training courses on offer

www.ippf.org.uk
Online version of the *Directory of Hormonal Contraception*, with names of (equivalent) pill brands used throughout the world

www.who.int/reproductive-health
WHO Medical Eligibility Criteria (WHOMEC) and new Practice Recommendations (WHOSPR)

www.rcog.org.uk
Evidence-based Royal College Guidelines on male and female sterilization, infertility and menorrhagia

www.ffprhc.org.uk
Includes detailed Faculty of FP guidance on numerous contraceptive topics and UK-adapted Medical Eligibility Criteria (UKMEC), also access to the invaluable *Journal of the Faculty of Family Planning and Reproductive Health Care*

www.nice.org.uk/guidance/CG30
Specific URL for valuable guidance from NICE on long-acting reversible contraceptives, 2005

www.fertilityuk.org
The fertility awareness and NFP service, including teachers available locally – a brilliant website, factual and non-sectarian

www.bashh.org
National guidelines for the management of all STIs and contact details for GUM clinics throughout the UK

www.fpa.org.uk
Patient information plus those essential leaflets! There is also an invaluable Helpline: 0845 310 1334

www.brook.org.uk
Similar to the FPA website but for under 25s; plus a really secure on-line enquiry service. Helpline: 0800 0185023

www.likeitis.org.uk
Reproductive health for lay persons by Marie Stopes. Brilliantly teenage-friendly and matter-of-factual

www.ruthinking.co.uk
Sex – are you thinking about it enough? Factual website that fully informs plus helps teens to access services in own local area. Supported by the Teenage Pregnancy Unit

www.teenagehealthfreak.com
FAQs as asked by teenagers, on all health subjects, not just reproductive health – from anorexia to zits!
Fourth of quartet of superb websites for young people

www.the-bms.org
Research-based advice about the menopause and hormone-replacement therapy (HRT)

www.ipm.org.uk
Website of the Institute of Psychosexual Medicine

www.basrt.org.uk
Website of the British Association for Sexual and Relationship Therapy; provides a list of therapists

www.relate.org.uk
Enter postcode to get nearest Relate centre for relationship counselling and psychosexual therapy. Many publications are also available

John Guillebaud's website regarding the Timecapsule plus 'Apology to the Future' project – and related sites:
www.ecotimecapsule.com
www. populationandsustainability.org
www.optimumpopulation.org
www. popconnect.org – source of the dramatic DVD 'Population Dots'
www.peopleandplanet.net

FURTHER READING

Filshie M, Guillebaud J. *Contraception: Science and Practice*. London: Butterworths, 1989.

Guillebaud J. *Contraception – Your Questions Answered*. Edinburgh: Churchill-Livingstone, 2004.

Guillebaud J. *Contraception* In: McPherson A, Waller D, eds. *Women's Health*, 5th edn. Oxford: Oxford University Press, 2003 [formerly *Women's Problems in General Practice*]

Kubba A, Sanfilippo J, Hampton N. *Contraception and Office Gynaecology: Choices in Reproductive Healthcare*. London: WB Saunders, 1999.

Potts M, Diggory P. *Textbook of Contraceptive Practice*. Cambridge: Cambridge University Press, 1983.

Sapire E. *Contraception and Sexuality in Health and Disease*. New York: McGraw-Hill, 1990.

WHO. *Medical Eligibility Criteria for Contraceptive Use (WHOMEC)*. Geneva: WHO, 2004.

WHO. *Selected Practice Recommendations for Contraceptive Use (WHOSPR)*. Geneva: WHO, 2005.

Or, more simply, visit the WHO website above; or that of the Faculty of FP to check any query with UKMEC, the UK adaptation of WHO guidance.

Background reading

(including titles for a general readership)

Cooper E, Guillebaud J. *Sexuality and Disability*. London: Radcliffe Medical Press, 1999.

Djerassi C. *This Man's Pill*. Oxford: Oxford University Press, 2001.

Ehrlich P, Ehrlich A. *The Population Explosion*. London: Arrow Books, 1991.

Guillebaud J. *The Pill*, 6th edn. Oxford: Oxford University Press, 2005.

Montford H, Skrine R. *Psychosexual Medicine Series 6. Contraceptive Care: Meeting Individual Needs*. London: Chapman & Hall, 1993.

Population Reports (various years to 2003) Excellent comprehensive reviews of the literature on developments in population, contraception and sterilisation: www.jhuccp.org.

Skrine R, Montford H. *Psychosexual Medicine – An Introduction*. London: Arnold, 2001.

Szarewski A, Guillebaud J. *Contraception – A User's Guide*, 3rd edn. Oxford: Oxford University Press, 2000.

Many more relevant book titles, as well as DVDs and useful patient leaflets concerning all methods, can be obtained by easy mail order from the UK Family Planning Association (FPA) and the International Planned Parenthood Federation (IPPF). See their websites above.

GLOSSARY

ALO	*Actinomyces*-like organisms
AMI	acute myocardial infarction
BBD	benign breast disease
BMI	body mass index
BNF	British National Formulary
BP	blood pressure
BTB	breakthrough bleeding
CGHFBC	Collaborative Group on Hormonal Factors in Breast Cancer
CIN	cervical intraepithelial neoplasia

COC	combined oral contraception/ive
COEC	combined oral emergency contraceptive
CPA	cyproterone acetate
CSM	Committee on the Safety of Medicines (UK)
CVS	cardiovascular system
DFFP	Diploma of the Faculty of Family Planning and Reproductive Health Care
DM	diabetes mellitus
DMPA	Depot medroxyprogesterone acetate (Depo-Provera)
DNA	deoxyribonucleic acid
DoH	Department of Health (now termed DH)
DSG	desogestrel
DSP	drospirenone
EC	emergency contraception
EE	ethinylestradiol
EVA	ethylene vinyl acetate
FFPRHC ⎫ Faculty of FP ⎭	Faculty of Family Planning and Reproductive Health Care
FAQ	frequently asked question
FGD 2003	Faculty Guidance Document 2003
FH	family history
FPA	Family Planning Association
FSH	follicle-stimulating hormone
GP	general practitioner
GSD	gestodene
GUM	genitourinary medicine
hCG	human chorionic gonadotrophin
HDL	high-density lipoprotein
HIV	human immunodeficiency virus
HPV	human papillomavirus
HRT	hormone-replacement therapy
HUS	haemolytic uraemic syndrome
INR	International Normalized Ratio – blood test used to control warfarin anticoagulant level
IPPF	International Planned Parenthood Federation
IUD	intrauterine device
IUS	intrauterine system
LAM	lactational amenorrhoea method
LARC	long-acting reversible contraceptive method
LCR	ligase chain reaction – ultrasensitive and specific test (e.g. for *Chlamydia*)
LMP	last menstrual period
LNG	levonorgestrel
MFFP	Membership of the Faculty of Family Planning and Reproductive Health Care

MHRA	Medicines and Healthcare Products Regulatory Agency
MPC	Margaret Pyke Centre
NET	norethisterone (termed norethindrone in the USA)
NETA	norethisterone acetate
NFP	natural family planning
NGM	norgestimate
NICE	National Institute for Health and Clinical Excellence
OR	odds ratio
PCOS	polycystic ovarian syndrome
PCR	polymerase chain reaction (like LCR, for ultrasensitive/specific tests)
PFI	pill-free interval
PID	pelvic inflammatory disease
PIL	Patient Information Leaflet
PMS	premenstrual syndrome
POEC	progestogen-only emergency contraceptive
POP	progestogen-only pill
RCGP	Royal College of General Practitioners
RCN	Royal College of Nursing
RCOG	Royal College of Obstetricians and Gynaecologists
RCT	randomized controlled trial
SHGB	sex-hormone-binding globulin
SLE	systemic lupus erythematosus
SPC	Summary of Product Characteristics (= Data Sheet)
SRE	sex and relationships education
STI	sexually transmitted infection
TIA	transient ischaemic attack
TTP	thrombotic thrombocytopenic purpura
UKMEC	adaptation by the Faculty of FP, for the UK, of WHO's Medical Eligibility Criteria for Contraceptive Use
UPSI	unprotected sexual intercourse
VTE	venous thromboembolism
VV	varicose veins
WHO	World Health Organization
WHOMEC	WHO Medical Eligibility Criteria for contraceptive use
WHOSPR	WHO's Selected Practice Recommendations for contraceptive use

Index

Page numbers in *italics* indicate tables or figures.

abortion, induced
  DMPA injection after
    82
  Implanon insertion
    after 95
  intrauterine contra-
    ception after 121
  IUD removal 104
  oral contraception
    after *54, 75*
absorption, impaired
  57
abstinence, periodic *8,*
  140–2
acne 14, 59, 60
Actinomyces-like
  organisms (ALOs)
  109–11
age
  copper IUD
    effectiveness and
    101
  discontinuation of
    contraception
    147–8
  see also older
    women; young
    women
allergy, to condoms
  135–6
amenorrhoea
  climacteric 147, 148
  DMPA-induced 84,
    85, 89
  LNG-IUS users 113,
    115–16
  POP-induced 76, 77
  secondary 60–1,
    145–6
  starting oral
    contraceptives *54,*
    75

  see also lactational
    amenorrhoea
    method
anaemia 112, 114
analgesia, IUD/IUS
  insertion 123
anorexia nervosa 86,
  88
antibiotics
  (antimicrobials)
  COC interactions
    50–1, 52
  POP interactions 71
  prophylactic, IUD
    insertion 109, 129
anti-emetics 130
anti-epileptic drugs
  COC interactions 50,
    51
  see also enzyme-
    inducing drugs;
    epilepsy
antiphospholipid
  antibodies 32
antiretrovirals 50
anxiety 35, 59
arachis oil 135
arterial disease
  COCs and 26, 34
  DMPA 85, 87
  LNG-IUS 116
  POP 72, 74
arterial disease risk
  factors
  COC *30–1,* 32–3,
    34, 36, 146
  DMPA 87, 88
  Implanon 94
aura, migraine 39–40,
  41, 61
Avanti 134
azithromycin 109, 129

baby oil 134, 135
barbiturates 50
barrier methods
  134–40
BiNovum *12*
bleeding
  abnormal menstrual
    see menstrual
    bleeding, abnormal
  breakthrough *see*
    breakthrough
    bleeding
  IUD users 103–4,
    111–12
  unexplained genital
    tract 35, 73, 87,
    94, 118
  withdrawal 47–8, 49
bleeding tendency 88
blood pressure (BP)
  monitoring 62, 76,
    89
  see also
    hypertension
body mass index (BMI)
  27
  raised *see*
    obesity/overweight
body weight/mass
  COC choice and 58,
    59
  DMPA-induced gain
    84, 88–9
  Implanon efficacy
    and 91
  Implanon-induced
    gain 97
  POP effectiveness
    and 69
bone mineral density
  DMPA users 84,
    85–6

Implanon users 97
bosentan 71–2
breakthrough bleeding
(BTB), COC users
49–50, 53, 55, *56,*
56–7
breast biopsy,
premalignant
epithelial atypia 17,
35
breast cancer
COC-related risk
14–17, *15, 17*
in complete remission
37, 74, 88, 94
current 35, 116–17,
118, 127
DMPA and 80
family history 17, 37,
75
POP and 72
recent, not in
remission 73, 87,
94
breast disease, benign
(BBD) 17, 37
breastfeeding *see*
lactation
breast tenderness 58,
76
Brevinor *12*
British Association for
Sexual and
Relationship Therapy
2, 153

cancer
COC-related risks
14–20, *21*
DMPA-related risk
80
IUD and LNG-IUS
users 113
sex-steroid
dependent 35, 37,
74, 88, 94
*see also specific
types*
Canestan 135
cap *see* diaphragm
carbamazepine 50, 71
cardiovascular disease
see arterial disease
Cerazette 68, 77–9
contraindications
73–5, 79
DMPA injections and
82
drug interactions
71–2

indications 72–3, 78
lactation and 71
mechanism of
action/efficacy
77–8
missed pills 70, 132
overweight women
69
side effects 72, 76,
78–9
starting routines 75
cerebral haemorrhage
26, 34
cerebrovascular
accident *see* stroke
cervical cancer, COC
users 18
cervical intraepithelial
neoplasia (CIN) 18,
37
cervical smears 37, 63
Chlamydia trachomatis
6
IUD users 108
screening 109, 129
choice of methods 3, *4*
chorea 35
choriocarcinoma, COCs
and 19
chronic systemic
disease 37, 75, 94
ciclosporin 51
Cilest *12*
circulatory disease *see*
arterial disease;
venous
thromboembolism
clarithromycin 50–1
climacteric 147–9
clonazepam 51
coital history,
emergency
contraception 130
colorectal cancer 20
combined hormonal
contraception 11–67
combined oral
contraceptives
(COCs) 11–64
absolute
contraindications
33–6, 41
benefits versus risks
11–20, *21*
bicycling 50
blood level variations
56
choices 32–3
circulatory disease
and 20–6

DMPA injections and
82
DMPA-related
bleeding problems
84
drug interactions
50–3
effectiveness *8*
eligibility criteria
33–7
first-time users 32
follow-up 62–4
formulations *12*
Implanon-related
bleeding problems
96
intercurrent diseases
37–42
IUD/IUS insertion
121–2
mechanism of action
11
missed pills *43,*
43–5, *46,* 47,
131–2
named-patient
prescribing 151
older women 16, *29,*
33, 146–7, 148
pill-free interval (PFI)
and efficacy *43,*
43–50, 55
prescribing guidelines
26–33
previous failure 47
proprietary names
worldwide 151–2
Quick start 131,
145, 151
relative
contraindications
36–7, 38–9, 41–2
second choice
56–60
side effects 58
smokers *29, 30,*
32–3, 146
starting 53–5, *54*
stopping 60–2
tricycling *47,* 47–50
venous
thromboembolism
risk 20–5, *24, 25*
vomiting and
diarrhoea 47
combined oral
emergency
contraceptive (COEC)
124
condoms 135–7

COC users 55
effectiveness *8,* 135
female *8, 136,*
136–7
spermicides with
136, 140
unsafe vaginal
preparations 134,
135
confidentiality 5, 129
congenital
abnormalities, COC
risks 63
consultations, time
needed 1–2
contraceptive services,
Levels 1, 2 and 3 1
contraindications, WHO
classification system
7–10
copper intrauterine
devices *see*
intrauterine devices
(IUDs), copper
corticosteroid therapy
87, 88
co-trimoxazole 50–1
CuT 380Ag 101
Cyclogest 135
cyproterone acetate
(CPA) *12,* 60
cystitis, chronic 138

Dalacin cream 135
Dalkon Shield 105
Delfen foam 139
Depo-Provera *see*
depot
medroxyprogesterone
acetate
Depo-subQ provera
104 81
depot
medroxyprogesterone
acetate (DMPA)
80–9
administration 80–1
advantages and
indications 83
contraindications 87–8
counselling 88–9
drug interactions 81
effectiveness *8,* 81
follow-up 89
mechanism of action
81
older women 85, 86,
148
overdue injections
82–3, 133, 145

problems and
disadvantages
83–7
starting routines
81–2
subcutaneous 81
depression 37, 58
desogestrel (DSG)
COCs *12,* 32–3
POP *see* Cerazette
venous
thromboembolism
risk 21–3, *22,* 24
diabetes mellitus (DM)
arterial disease risk
26, *30*
COC prescribing
32–3, 36, 38
DMPA and 88
intrauterine
contraception 120
POP 73
Dianette *12,* 58, 60
diaphragm (cap)
137–9
arcing spring 138
effectiveness *8,*
137–8
spermicides with *8,*
137, 139
unsafe vaginal
preparations 134,
135
vault or cervical 138
diarrhoea, COC users
47, 57
diuretics, potassium-
sparing 51
DMPA *see* depot
medroxyprogesterone
acetate
domperidone 130
Double-Dutch approach
6, 118
doxycycline 84, 96
drospirenone 51, 59
see also Yasmin
drug interactions
COC 50–3
DMPA 81
Implanon 92
levonorgestrel
emergency
contraception 126
POP 71–2
Dubin–Johnson
syndrome 35
dysmenorrhoea, intra-
uterine contraception
114, 120

E45 135
Ecostatin 135
ectopic pregnancy
copper IUD users
103, 111
emergency
contraception and
130
LNG-IUS users 115
previous 74, 83, 93,
119
effectiveness/failure
rates 7, *8*
eligibility criteria,
medical 7–10
emergency
contraception (EC)
124–33
breastfeeding and
71, 127, 132
Chlamydia screening
109
copper IUDs 100,
102, 119, 124,
125, 127–9
counselling and
management
129–31
follow-up 131
levonorgestrel
progestogen-only
see levonorgestrel
emergency
contraceptive
LNG-IUS and 117
methods 124, *125*
missed COCs 45,
131–2
missed POPs 70,
132
named-patient
prescribing 151
special indications
131–3
starting COC after
54, 131, 145
endocarditis 119
endometrial
ablation/resection
120
endometrial cancer 20,
80
endometriosis 14, 49,
83, 120
enzyme-inducing drugs
COC and 37, 50,
51, 52–3
DMPA and 81
Evra and 66
Implanon and 92

levonorgestrel
  emergency
    contraception 126
  NuvaRing and 67
  POP interactions 71,
    74
epilepsy
  COCs 49, 51, 52–3
  DMPA 83
  LNG-IUS 114
erythema multiforme
  83
erythromycin 50–1
estrogen
  COC formulations
    12
  deficiency, DMPA
    users 85–6
  DMPA-related
    bleeding problems
    84
  drug interactions 49,
    50
  Implanon-related
    bleeding problems
    96
ethinylestradiol (EE)
  COCs 11, 12
  DMPA-related
    bleeding problems
    84
  Evra patches 65
  NuvaRing 66
  venous
    thromboembolism
    risk 21–3, 22
ethosuximide 51
ethylene vinyl acetate
  (EVA) 90, 91
etonogestrel 66
  implants see
    Implanon
etynodiol diacetate 68
Eugynon 12, 58
Evra patch 8, 65–6,
  148
Ez-On condom 134, 136

factor V Leiden 27
Faculty of Family
  Planning and
  Reproductive Health
  Care (FFPRHC) 2,
  9, 122–3, 152
failure
  rates/effectiveness
  7, 8
Family Planning
  Association (FPA) 3,
  53–5, 152

Femcap 138
Femidom 136, 136–7
Femodene 12, 53
Femodette 12
Femulen 68
fertility, return of
  COC users 63–4
  DMPA users 84, 89
  LNG-IUS users 113,
    115
  POP users 77
fertility awareness
  methods 140–2
fibroids, uterine 120
Flexi-T 300 99, 102,
  103
Flexi-T 380 99, 102,
  103
fluid retention 58, 59
follicle-stimulating
  hormone (FSH) 72,
  77, 147, 148
Fraser guidelines 5

gallstones 37
genitourinary medicine
  (GUM) clinic 109
gestational trophoblastic
  disease see
  trophoblastic disease,
  gestational
gestodene (GSD)
  COCs 12, 32–3
  venous
    thromboembolism
    and 21–3, 22, 24
Gilbert's disease 35
griseofulvin 50
GyneFix 99, 102–3,
  120
Gyno-Daktarin 135
Gynol II jelly 139
Gyno-Pevaryl 135

haemolytic uraemic
  syndrome (HUS) 35,
  36
headaches
  COC users 49, 55,
    61, 62
  migraine 39–40
heart disease
  COCs 34
  DMPA 85
  IUD/IUS 119
  POPs 73, 78
hepatitis 35
hepatocellular cancer,
  primary 18
high altitude 34, 36

hirsutism 59, 60
HIV
  infection, LNG-IUS
    use 119
  prevention of
    transmission 135,
    137
  spermicide use and
    140
hormone replacement
  therapy (HRT) 147,
  148
  plus LNG-IUS 114,
    117, 147
human papillomavirus
  (HPV) 18
hyperkalaemia 51
hyperlipidaemia, familial
  88
hyperprolactinaemia 37
hypertension
  arterial disease risk
    26, 31
  COC-induced 38, 62
  COC prescribing 35,
    38–9
  essential 39
  POP 73
  pregnancy-induced
    39

ibuprofen 123
ideal contraceptive 6–7
immobility, COC use
  and 29, 34, 61
immunosuppression 118
Implanon 90
  contraindications
    93–4
  counselling and
    follow-up 95–6
  drug interactions 92
  effectiveness 8, 91
  indications 93
  insertion 90, 91, 95
  mechanism of action
    91
  reversibility and
    removal problems
    92
  side effects 93,
    96–7
implants 90–7
  effectiveness 8
  see also Implanon
infants, POP dose 71
inflammatory bowel
  disease 37
information leaflets 3,
  53–5

injectables 80–97
Institute of
Psychosexual
Medicine 2, 153
International Planned
Parenthood
Federation (IPPF)
151–2
intracranial
hypertension, benign
35
intrauterine
contraception
98–123
intrauterine devices
(IUDs), copper
98–113, *99*
advantages 99–100
analgesia for
insertion 123
banded 99, *99*, 100,
101
cancer risk 113
choice and
effectiveness
100–3
contraindications
118–20, 129
counselling and
follow-up 122
duration of use
112–13
effectiveness *8*
emergency
contraception *see
under* emergency
contraception
expulsion 103, 132
insertion
arrangements
108–9
insertion timing
121–2
insertion training
122–3
lost threads 104–5,
106
malpositioning 103,
112
mechanism of action
100
named-patient
prescribing 151
pelvic inflammatory
disease 103,
105–9, *107*
perforation 103, 105
problems and
disadvantages
103–12

removal 132
ischaemic heart
disease 34

Jadelle 90
jaundice, cholestatic
34–5

Kawasaki disease 34
KY Jelly 134

lactation (breastfeeding)
COCs 35, *54*
DMPA injections 82
emergency
contraception 71,
127, 132
Implanon insertion
95
POPs 70–1, 72, *75*
lactational amenorrhoea
method (LAM) 70,
142, *143*
lamotrigine 51
lansoprazole 51
Lea's Shield 138
Levonelle 1500 *see*
levonorgestrel
emergency
contraceptive
levonorgestrel (LNG)
COCs *12*, 32–3
POP 68
venous
thromboembolism
risk 20–3, *22*,
24–5
levonorgestrel
emergency
contraceptive (LNG
EC) 124, *125*,
125–7
advanced provision
133
advantages 126
contraindications
127
counselling and
management
129–31
effectiveness *8*, 126
enzyme-inducer
therapy and 126
follow up 131
mechanism of action
125
side effects 130
special indications
131–3
levonorgestrel-releasing

intrauterine system
(LNG-IUS) 98,
113–19
advantages and
indications 114–15
analgesia for
insertion 123
contraindications
116–17, 118–20
counselling and
follow-up 122
duration of use 117
ectopic pregnancy
111
effectiveness *8*, 113
insertion timing
121–2
insertion training
122–3
method of action
113–14, *114*
named-patient
prescribing 151
plus HRT 114, 117,
147
problems and
disadvantages
115–16
licensed products,
unlicensed use
150–1
lipid disorders,
atherogenic 34
liver disease 34–5, 74,
88, 94, 116, 127
liver tumours 18, 35,
116, 120
Load 375 *99*
local anaesthesia
implant
insertion/removal
91, 92
IUD/IUS insertion
123
Loestrin 20/30 *12*, 48,
58
Logynon *12*, 48
Lomexin 135
long-acting reversible
contraceptive
methods (LARCs) 1,
3, 4, *4*, 90
lubricants, vaginal 134,
135
Lunelle *8*

Marvelon *12*, 58, 59,
60
medroxyprogesterone
acetate, depot *see*

depot medroxyprogesterone acetate
mefenamic acid 112, 123
melanoma, malignant 37
menopause
  discontinuation of contraception 147–9
  POP users 77
menorrhagia, LNG-IUS 114, 120
menstrual bleeding, abnormal
  COC benefits 13
  DMPA users 84–5, 89
  Implanon and 93, 94, 96
  IUD users 103–4, 111–12
  LNG-IUS 114, 115–16
  POP users 72, 75–6, 78–9
menstrual cycle
  emergency contraception and 130
  first DMPA injection 82
  IUD/IUS insertion 121
  starting COC *54*
  starting POP *75*
Mercilon *12*
methods of contraception
  choice 3, *4*
  ideal 6–7
  relative effectiveness 7, *8*
Microgynon *12*, 45, 53
  as second choice pill 58
  tricycling 48
  venous thromboembolism risk 24–5
Micronor 68
mifepristone 124
migraine 39–42
  with aura 39–40, 41, 61
  COC prescribing 34, 41–2
  differential diagnosis 42

POP 73
  stroke risk 26, *31*, 39
minipill *see* progestogen-only pill
Minulet *12*
Mirena *see* levonorgestrel-releasing intrauterine system
miscarriage
  DMPA injections 82
  IUD users 103, 104
  oral contraception after *54*, *75*
modafinil 50
morning-after pill 124
Multiload Cu375 *99*
Multiload IUDs 102
myocardial infarction, acute (AMI) 26, *30–1*, 33

named-patient prescribing 150–1
National Institute for Clinical Excellence (NICE) 1, 152
natural family planning (NFP) methods *8*, 140–2
nevirapine 50
Nizoral 135
nonoxinol-9 135–6, 137, 140
norelgestromin 65
norethisterone (NET)
  COCs *12*, 32–3
  enanthate (injectable) 80–1
  POPs 68
  venous thromboembolism risk 21, *22*
norgestimate (NGM) *12*, 23
Norgeston 68
Noriday 68
Norimin *12*, 48
Norinyl-1 *12*, 52
Noristerat 80–1
Norplant *8*, 91
  side effects 96, 97
Nova-T 380 *99*, 102
nulliparous women, intrauterine contraception 101, 119, 129
nurse prescribers 150–1

NuvaRing *8*, 66–7
Nystan cream 135

obesity/overweight
  COC prescribing *31*, 34, 36
  COC risks *28*
  DMPA and 88
  Evra 65
  Implanon 91
  POPs 69, 73, 78
older women 146–9
  arterial disease risk *31*
  COCs 16, *29*, 33, 146–7, 148
  copper IUDs 101, 109
  diaphragm 137–8
  discontinuation of contraception 147–9
  DMPA 85, 86, 148
  LNG-IUS 117, 147, 148
  POPs 73, 77, 148
  spermicidal products 139, 148
oligo/amenorrhoea
  COC use 37
  LNG-IUS users 115–16
  POP users 72, 78–9
  see also amenorrhoea; menstrual bleeding, abnormal
Ortho-Crème 139
Orthoform pessaries 139
Ortho-Gynest 135
osteoporosis 85, 86, 87
otosclerosis 37
ovarian cancer, COC users 20
ovarian cysts, functional 74, 76, 83, 94, 116
overweight *see* obesity/overweight
Ovranette *12*, 48
Ovysmen *12*
oxcarbazepine 50

pain, IUD users 103–4, 111–12
pancreatitis 35
parents, under-16s 5
pelvic infections
  current 118

past history 119, 130
pelvic inflammatory disease (PID)
copper IUD users 103, 105–9, *107*
LNG-IUS users 115
pemphigoid gestationis 35
penicillamine 120
Persona 141–2, *142*
petroleum jelly 135
pharmacists, emergency contraception 129–30
phenytoin 50
polycystic ovary syndrome (PCOS) 32, 59
porphyria 35, 73, 74, 87, 88, 94, 127
postcoital contraception *see* emergency contraception
postpartum period 145–6
COCs 35, 36, *54*
DMPA injections 82
Implanon insertion 95
intrauterine contraception 120, 121
POPs *75*
potassium-sparing diuretics 51
practice nurses 2
pregnancy
contraindicating contraception 35, 73, 87, 94, 118
criteria for excluding 144
ectopic *see* ectopic pregnancy
emergency contraception and 127
IUD users 103, 104, 105
tests 144, 145, 146
pregnancy-induced hypertension 39
premenstrual syndrome (PMS) 49, 59, 114
primidone 50
progestogen-only emergency contraceptive pill *see*

levonorgestrel emergency contraceptive
progestogen-only pill (POP) 68–79
contraindications 73–5
counselling and supervision 75–7
DMPA injections and 82
drug interactions 71–2
effectiveness *8,* 69
indications 72–3
lactation and 70–1
mechanism of action 68–9
missed pills 69–70, 132
named-patient prescribing 151
older women 73, 77, 148
risks and disadvantages 72
side effects 72, 75–6
starting COC after *54*
starting routines *75*
progestogens
COCs *12,* 32–3
implants 90–7
venous thromboembolism risk 20–3, *22*
prostheses 120
prosthetic valve replacement 119
prothrombotic states 34
proton-pump inhibitors 51
pulmonary hypertension 34, 71–2, 73, 78, 119

Quick start 131, 145, 151

rape 119, 129
rifabutin 50, 52, 53, 81
rifampicin 50, 51, 52, 53, 71, 81
ritonavir 50
Rotor syndrome 35
RU486 124

Seasonale 48
seborrhoea 59

sex and relationships education (SRE) 3–5
sexual abuse 5
sexual assault 129
sexual history 6, 108–9
sexual intercourse, unprotected (UPSI) 124
time after 126, 127, 128, 132
see also emergency contraception
sexually transmitted infections (STIs)
current 118
IUD users 107–9
LNG-IUS and 118
protection against 6–7, 134
women at high risk 119
see also pelvic inflammatory disease
sickle cell disease/trait 37, 73, 83
smokers
COC *29, 30,* 32–3, 146
POP 73
risks 26, 27
spermicides *8,* 139–40
with condoms 136, 140
with diaphragms *8,* 137, 139
sponge *8,* 139, 148
sterilization
female 3, 134
male 134
Stevens–Johnson syndrome 35
St John's Wort 50, 126
stroke
COC-related risk 26
migraine-related risk 26, *31,* 39
risk factors *30–1*
Sturge–Weber syndrome 35
subarachnoid haemorrhage 26
subfertility, suspected 119
Sultrin 135
surgery, major or leg 34, 61, 73, 78
Synphase *12*

systemic lupus erythematosus (SLE) 35

teratogenicity 83, 104, 130
termination of pregnancy *see* abortion, induced
tetracycline 52
thrombophilias 27–32, *28*, 34
thrombotic thrombocytopenic purpura (TTP) 35
thrush 36
Today sponge 139
topiramate 50
toxaemia of pregnancy 39
training 2
   diaphragm fitting 138–9
   Implanon use 91, 92
   IUD/IUS insertion 122–3
tranexamic acid 112
transdermal combined hormonal contraception 65–6
   see also Evra patch
transient ischaemic attacks (TIAs) 34, 42, 61
transvaginal combined hormonal contraception 66–7
Triadene *12*
Tri-Minulet *12*
Trinordiol *12*
TriNovum *12*, 48
trophoblastic disease, gestational
   COC after 19, 35, *54*
   DMPA after 88
   emergency contraception 127
   Implanon 94
   intrauterine contraception 117, 118

POP after 74
T-Safe Cu 380A 100, 101, 103
   duration of use 112
   ectopic pregnancy and 111
T-Safe Cu 380A QL *99*, 100
TT 380 Slimline *99*, 100
tuberculosis 52–3

UK Medical Eligibility Criteria (UKMEC) 9–10
under-16s 4–6
Uniject 81
unlicensed use of licensed products 150–1
UT 380 Short *99*, 102, 103
uterus
   congenital abnormalities 120
   distorted cavity 118, 120
   perforation 103, 105, 120

vaginal preparations 134, 135
valproate 51
varicose veins *29*
Vaseline 135
venous disease, COC prescribing 34, 36
venous thromboembolism (VTE)
   COC discontinuation 61
   COC prescribing 32–3, 34
   COC-related risk 20–5, *24*, *25*
   DMPA and 83
   hereditary predispositions 27, *28*

Implanon and 93, 94
LNG-IUS 116
personal history 27, *28*, 34
POP and 73, 74
risk factors 27–32, *28–9*
vigabatrin 51
vomiting
   COCs and 47, 55, 57
   emergency contraception and 128, 130

warfarin 88, 126
weaning, POP users 71
websites 152–3
weight *see* body weight/mass
Wilson's disease 119
Witepsol-based preparations 135
withdrawal bleeding 47–8, 49
withdrawal method *8*
World Health Organization (WHO) classification of contraindications 7–10
   Medical Eligibility Criteria (WHOMEC) 9–10, 152
   Selected Practice Recommendations (WHOSPR) 9, 144, 152

Yasmin *12*
   contraindications 35
   drug interactions 51
   uses 58, 59, 60
young women 3–6
   under 16 years 4–6
   DMPA 86
   intrauterine contraception 119